The Art of
Cosmic Vision

The Art of Cosmic Vision

Practices for Improving Your Eyesight

Mantak Chia
and
Robert T. Lewanski

Destiny Books
Rochester, Vermont • Toronto, Canada

Destiny Books
One Park Street
Rochester, Vermont 05767
www.DestinyBooks.com

Destiny Books is a division of Inner Traditions International

Originally published in Thailand in 2008 by Universal Healing Tao Publications under the title *Cosmic Vision: Art of Improving Vision Naturally*

Library of Congress Cataloging-in-Publication Data
Chia, Mantak, 1944–
 [Cosmic vision]
 The art of cosmic vision : practices for improving your eyesight / Mantak Chia and Robert T. Lewanski.
  p. cm.
 Originally published: Cosmic vision. Thailand : Universal Healing Tao Publications, 2008.
 Includes bibliographical references and index.
 ISBN 978-1-59477-293-1 (pbk.)
 1. Eye—Care and hygiene. 2. Visual acuity. 3. Holistic medicine. 4. Taoists.
5. Medicine, Ayurvedic. I. Lewanski, Robert T. II. Title.
 RE51.C53 2010
 617.7—dc22

                                                              2009048199

Printed and bound in the United States by Berryville Graphics

10 9 8 7 6 5 4 3 2 1

Text design and layout by Priscilla Baker
This book was typeset in Janson, with Futura and Present used as display typefaces

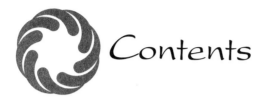

Contents

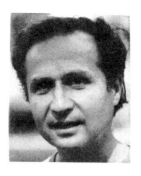

This book is dedicated to Robert Zuraw, who made its publication possible through his research and practice. Bob studied with Helen Tulmich, an instructor in the Dr. Bates-Corbett school of visual education from 1961 to 1963. He also studied with Dr. Sasaki, a natural eye doctor from Ann Arbor, Michigan. From 1964 to 1966 he was a sergeant nurse in the Army in Vietnam, for thirteen months in Saigon. He assisted surgeons in major operations with medical instruments and emergency causality readiness. He graduated with honors from the Career Academy, School of Famous Television and Radio Broadcasters in Washington, D.C. He was personally instructed by the well-known broadcasters John Cameron Swayze, Robert St. John, and Al Michaels for two years, 1968 to 1969. He was president of the Michigan Vegetarian Society from 1967 to 1988.

In 1985 he studied with Dr. Shen Wang in the Art of Chinese Flying Crane Chi Kung Yoga Meditation. In 1987, he became a Certified Instructor in the Tien Tao Chi Kung System of the Chinese National Chi Kung Institute at the culmination of a one-year course in Esoteric Chi Kung exercises and meditation. In 1990, Robert studied with Zen Taoist Master Venerable Hyunoong Sunim, a Buddhist monk from the mountains of Korea. From Master Hyunoong Sunim, he learned the Five-Element Body Typing System, Taoist nutritional and herbal medicine, and Taoist breathing exercises, which helped him to overcome a severe energy blockage. He learned the Taoist Sun-Do meditation and Taoist yoga techniques, Do-In Self-Massage, and Body Typing Energy Analysis. Bob passed away December 14, 2006, and is missed by hundreds of students for his kindness, knowledge, and generosity.

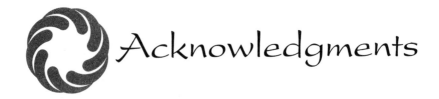 Acknowledgments

We extend our gratitude to all the great teachers of natural eye training throughout history who have given us hope and insight into holistic health and vision training practices. We thank all the wise doctors and teachers who, over the years, helped us formulate the principles of exercise, diet, herbal remedies, body typing, and Chi Kung that went into the development of this program for perfect eyesight.

We offer special thanks to our parents who brought us here for this purpose, and who gave us the freedom to grow and learn on our own. Thanks to our good friends and students who have supported us in our endeavors.

We wish to thank the following people for their assistance in producing the earlier editions of this book: Jason Schofield, Joe Alexander, Peter Klco, and W. U. Wei.

We also acknowledge and dedicate this book to all those sovereign, free-thinking individuals throughout the world who are seeking higher wisdom and the freedom to express their creativity in natural and spiritual ways.

Above all, we are grateful and thankful for the Creator of Heaven and Earth who gave us this opportunity to discover, learn, and teach these principles, so that others may also benefit from them.

Putting the Art of Cosmic Vision into Practice

The practices described in this book have been used successfully for thousands of years by Taoists trained by personal instruction. Readers should not undertake the practice without receiving personal transmission and training from a certified instructor of the Universal Tao, since certain of these practices, if done improperly, may cause injury or result in health problems. This book is intended to supplement individual training by the Universal Tao and to serve as a reference guide for these practices. Anyone who undertakes these practices on the basis of this book alone, does so entirely at his or her own risk.

The meditations, practices, and techniques described herein are *not* intended to be used as an alternative or substitute for professional medical treatment and care. If any readers are suffering from illnesses based on mental or emotional disorders, an appropriate professional health care practitioner or therapist should be consulted. Such problems should be corrected before you start training.

Neither the Universal Tao nor its staff and instructors can be responsible for the consequences of any practice or misuse of the information contained in this book. If the reader undertakes any exercise without strictly following the instructions, notes, and warnings, the responsibility must lie solely with the reader.

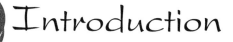

Introduction

Discover the Real Secrets of How You Can Attain Perfect Eyesight without Glasses or Surgery

The world today is full of men and women who endure unnecessary suffering because of poor eyesight. They think that glasses will cure or eliminate the conditions responsible for eye troubles. But glasses are nothing more than eye crutches. The real help must come from other sources. In the case of the eyes, it is exercise and corrective eye habits. Natural eye science offers normal vision through a simple system of eye correction.

Yes, both of us writing this book have quit wearing eyeglasses and now we both see perfectly. You too can stop wearing glasses and regain normal vision. You no longer need to suffer with unnecessary eye problems. Not only that, you will be able to see better than ever before.

Think of it. After being a slave to cumbersome glasses for years, you can discard your glasses forever. What a sense of accomplishment and satisfaction! Building up the strength of your eyes can be an enjoyable process—and not a very lengthy one. In most cases, a few short months of self-treatment in the correct eye exercise techniques can improve your vision tremendously.

A WONDERFUL STORY OF EYESIGHT REGAINED

Over thirty years ago, Robert Zuraw had a most trying experience with his eyes. Without his glasses, he was legally blind. Eye doctors gave him no hope of ever improving his vision or discarding his glasses. But he was not yet ready to throw in the towel. He was a fighter—a real street fighter in his youth—and his determined willpower kicked in. The idea of wearing glasses was intolerable, absolutely annoying. He knew there had to be someone who could help him. Always willing to back up his theories by experimenting upon himself, he immediately sought and eventually found natural eye improvement specialists, and started upon a course of natural eye treatment that he fully believed would help him.

With the help of natural eye trainers, plus books and eye courses from around the world, he entered into a period of research and experiment during which his vision zoomed from 20–600 to 20–20 and continued to improve annually until his death in 2006. The results were so entirely satisfactory that he associated himself with two of the few really great natural eye specialists. Through their collaboration, and his incredible reversal of advanced myopia, a remarkable new scientific system of eye training has risen, like a phoenix from the ashes. This system will quickly enable you to train the muscles of your eyes so that you too can make them work properly at all times, without effort or strain.

We have written *The Art of Cosmic Vision* to share the secrets of perfect eyesight with you. It will enable you to learn the real truth about how the eyes work. If you already wear glasses, find out how you can discard them. If you do not wear glasses, but feel that your sight is failing, then find out how a few minutes each day can assure you perfect sight without the use of glasses. If you are a parent you can learn how to save your children from the scourge of poor eyesight—how you can save them from the slavery of eyeglasses. Learn how thousands of other people have regained normal vision.

The Art of Cosmic Vision represents more than thirty-five years of study and research on improving eyesight naturally, without glasses or surgery. This book will tell you about the powers hidden within you that you can use to improve your vision far beyond the average. It will teach you the wonders and healing powers of the human eye, brain, nervous system, and body and explain why you were designed by the Creator to see perfectly without glasses. The book is loaded with never-before-revealed secrets of the eye-brain connection, and several exercises, including the Egyptian Black Dot Technique, that can improve your vision within minutes.

The Art of Cosmic Vision will show you just what is wrong with your eyes and how to overcome poor vision . . . sometimes within days! Cancel your eyeglass or eye surgery appointment until you read and practice the invaluable, result-producing information in this book, information that has been pronounced priceless by thousands.

"LET THERE BE LIGHT"

With all our advanced technology, we still know little about light and its greatest use—that of helping eyes to see clearly with the minimum of effort. But now we are beginning to learn some very interesting and fundamental facts about the relation of light to sight. To appreciate its full significance, however, we must first understand the conditions under which our eyes have developed.

In the beginning of the human race humans were creatures of the outdoors and their day extended only from dawn to dusk. Dependence on the sun for light continued for countless centuries. Then came "improvements" of fuel oil lanterns and candles. As civilization advanced, lighting methods advanced slowly with it. After oil lamps came gas lighting. It was not until Edison discovered how to produce light electrically within a bottle that the world made any marked progress in lighting.

Primitive humans used their eyes outdoors under very high intensities of light—intensities hundreds of times greater than we find indoors today. When the sun went down their tasks were ended for the day. They closed their eyes and went to sleep. During the day they used their eyes for distant seeing—hunting, fishing, foraging— and the most menial of seeing tasks. Very little close vision work was performed. Even by Abraham Lincoln's time, very few people studied or sewed or read as we do—far into the night.

Modern civilization has completely changed all this. We have lightly tossed aside the fact that our eyes had been developing for hundreds of thousands of years. For all that time, they were developing according to four principles of nature:

1. Distance seeing
2. Tremendous quantities of light to aid vision
3. A relatively short day
4. Easy visual tasks

In the last few seconds on the clock of time we have taken liberties with all four of nature's principles: we have substituted close seeing indoors, extremely low levels of lighting, a much longer day, and abnormally severe eye-straining tasks.

The eye is a marvelous organ, but not so remarkable that it is able to adapt itself to the severe change we have imposed upon it. Perhaps that is why so much eye trouble is prevalent today.

Cats can see in the dark. But your eyes and a child's eyes were never intended to do close seeing in anything but adequate light. Nature certainly never intended that we should use our eyes the way we do—for reading books, playing games, using computers, sewing, or other close work, in half light. It is no wonder that 75 percent of all people over thirty years of age have impaired vision! Even many of grade school children have defective eyesight and require glasses or contacts. What they really need is less close work, better lighting, and more outdoor activity.

Certainly, something is radically wrong when we try to read or perform office work under poor light. It is not only a matter of eyestrain. It is a matter of needlessly using up untold quantities of nervous energy. The statement has been made that the office worker who uses his or her eyes all day under inadequate light may be actually more tired at night than the person who spends all day laying bricks or building a house. This indicates quite clearly that it does take energy to see and that seeing consumes energy just as definitely as shoveling snow or washing a car.

Suppose you drive your car for fifty miles on a bright sunny day over a straight highway. At the end of the ride you notice no particular exhaustion. But drive the same car on the same road at night, in a fog—you will know that you have been doing some work. The only difference is in the lighting. You have gripped that wheel, tensed your muscles, strained your whole body; you have used up a tremendous amount of nervous energy just trying to see.

Years ago, scientific studies were conducted to measure human energy consumed in the process of seeing. Dozens of people were chosen for special laboratory tests. In one, each subject was seated in a comfortable chair and asked to read page after page of a well-printed book. As the subject read, his hand rested on a button, which he was requested to press at the end of each page. This was a means adapted for concealing the *real* purpose of the button.

What the subject did not know was that he was unconsciously recording the development of nervous muscular tension produced by the reading. It was found that the average pressure unknowingly exerted upon the key was 63 grams when the reading was done under very poor light. This pressure dropped to 43 grams when the illumination was raised. In other words, the drain of nervous energy, as indicated by tension in the hand, was decreased by a third with the use of more light. Such tests explain why poor lighting at the office or work place is a major cause of fatigue and tiredness. Poor lighting and eyestrain saps much of our energy.

Typists, bookkeepers, printers, mechanics, and other people who use their eyes constantly are often unnecessarily fatigued before the day is over. Proper lighting can do much to ward off this fatigue and to help them accomplish their tasks with greater ease, accuracy, and speed. Some interesting conclusions have been reached as a result of these tests:

The pupil of the eye becomes smaller with age; consequently, there is need for more light as we age.

If a child has to hold a book closer to his eyes than 13 or 14 inches, the probability is that he needs eyeglasses or better lighting or both.

The eyes readily adjust themselves to a variety of conditions, but will weaken under poor lighting and strain.

Three times as much light is required for reading a newspaper as for reading a well-printed book.

Good lighting or outdoor light helps defective eyes and prevents normal eyes from weakening.

Detailed close work, such as sewing, watch repair, electronic repair work, surgery, and so on, is harder on the eyes than reading; therefore, much more light is needed.

Reading in bed is usually hard on the eyes, not only because of poor posture, but also because of inadequate and improper lighting. By correcting both conditions, the strain on the eyes is materially decreased.

Reading when the page is brightly illuminated and rest of the room is comparatively dark often causes unnecessary eyestrain and fatigue. Some of the light should go to the walls and ceiling to bring more light in and lessen eyestrain.

Now you want to know what you can do about it. You want to know how you can light your home to conserve your eyesight and energy. The requirements for lighting the average room where most of your eye work is done are as follows:

1. Enough light—one or two 200-watt bulbs or full spectrum lights
2. Proper distribution of the light around the room
3. Absence of glare on the page or work surface, with a reflected glow upward

Many books have been written on eyesight improvement and holistic health. However, a rare experience awaits you. Never before has a book been written that encompasses the health relationship between body, mind, and eyes. In Eastern cultures and religions the body, mind, and spirit are not separated. The person and the whole of existence are seen as one: what affects one part affects the whole. Eastern cultures and religions have practiced and taught a holistic view of health and the universe for thousands of years. The word *health* means to be whole and complete in body, mind, and spirit. This holistic view of life also includes the eyes, which are considered to be "the windows of the soul."

Here in this inspiring and informative book you will discover long-lost formulas and secret eye health teachings. These secrets have been taught by masters, holistic health practitioners, eye specialists, and eye doctors throughout the ages. You will discover how the three main ayurvedic body types—air (*vata*), fire (*pitta*), and water (*kapha*)—affect health and eyesight. Your health and vision can improve rapidly when you consume the correct foods for your individual constitutional body type. Discovering and applying this information can make the difference between dim failing eyesight and poor health, and unlimited zestful and youthful vitality. Perfect eyesight can be retained far into advanced age. This is no idle boast. We challenge you to prove and test these teachings for yourself. Take nothing for granted. "Prove all things, hold fast to that which is true."

To further improve your eyesight, we have included special Chi Kung energy exercises and Do-In Self-Massage techniques designed to boost your internal energy, improve glandular function, enhance hormones, and circulate rich red oxygen-filled blood to your eyes and brain. The Chi Kung movements are fun and easy to do and they will help you to think, feel, and look young again. You'll also discover how to stay grounded, centered, and balanced, to remain strong and alert, and develop your intuition, intelligence, and physical strength. Plus, you will learn about special herbs, tonics, and foods to detoxify your liver and cleanse your body, which helps to improve vision.

You'll be introduced to proven principles, the personal application of which can literally transform your vision, if you practice them persistently and consistently. All of the eye, health, and Chi Kung techniques have been tested and proven safe for both the beginner and the advanced student, young or old. You can progress as far as you wish to go in regaining or maintaining superb vision, health, beauty, strength, and fitness.

Every day that you apply these powerful eye and health techniques, you will build and improve your life. Why not start today, right now, and decide that you too can benefit by these wonderful restorative methods? Discover for yourself what a dramatic transformation they will create. Then let others marvel at the results you have achieved.

By following these practices, life will take on a new meaning for you. You will begin to spiral upward to a new awareness and a higher sense of self. Because of your newfound purpose in life, arising from increased wisdom, understanding, knowledge, and practice, your vision will begin to improve. You will begin to "see" things clearly, not only visually, but also spiritually and intuitively.

You are about to embark on a sacred journey: a vision quest into the world of crystal clear eyesight, health rejuvenation, and unlimited energy. It is a journey you have to take all by yourself. You and only *you* must acquire the knowledge, wisdom, and understanding to apply these teachings to your life. Nothing in life is free. There is always a price to pay through effort or sweat equity. However, the rewards are satisfying: freedom from bothersome eyeglasses or contacts; saving thousands of dollars over a lifetime of purchasing eyewear; freedom from disease; crystal-clear vision; and bountiful health and energy. Isn't this worth working for?

Knowledge is power. By applying the knowledge of this book, you too can improve your vision and maintain it, with clarity and power, for a lifetime. May you attain the perfect eyesight and super health you are seeking! Turn the page to chapter 1 and begin your vision and health improvement quest today.

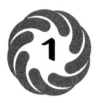

The Miracle of Perfect Eyesight

THE TRUTH ABOUT THE EYES

How clear is your vision? Can you see the world without blurring or distortion? The so-called normal eye can easily read the 20-foot line on the Snellen Eye Test Chart at 20 feet away—this is called 20–20 vision and is generally regarded as good vision. However, there is no limit to how much a person's vision can be improved beyond the 20–20 range. A person with above average eyesight can easily read the 10-foot line (smallest line on the Snellen Eye Test Chart) at 20 feet away, which means they have 20–10 vision. We have seen people who can read the 10 foot line at 50 to 60 feet away—60–10 vision! This is called "telescopic vision." There is also no limit to reading microscopically small print—this capacity is known as "microscopic vision."

Healthy eyes are a marvel of nature's creation. We are all walking, talking, seeing miracles. The sages say human beings are "solidified sunlight," or "trails of light," because our eyesight and our very life are totally dependent on the solar orb! We would all become blind without the healing rays of sunlight upon our retina. Sunlight also gives us natural vitamin D for healthy skin and eyes.

A QUICK LESSON IN EYE ANATOMY

The normal healthy eye is almost spherical and is made up of three layers of tissue:

1. The outer layer, or sclera
2. The middle layer, or choroid
3. The inner layer, or retina (fig. 1.1)

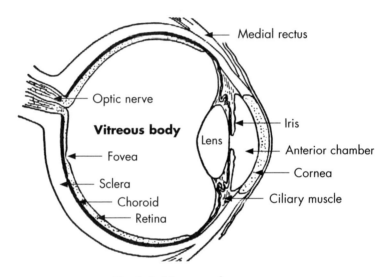

Fig. 1.1. Diagram of an eye

The first or sclerotic layer is opalescent. Its center is transparent and is called the cornea. Light comes through the cornea. Behind the cornea, the second layer, or choroid, is visible. It contains tiny blood vessels that transport blood to and from the eyes. The choroid layer also contains the iris, with the pupil in its center. Right behind the iris is the crystalline lens; the lens absorbs light as it passes through the pupil and focuses it upon the retina.

The choroid layer forms in rolls around the crystalline lens and is known as the ciliary process. Located here is the ciliary muscle; it is connected with the crystalline lens by a tiny ligament and controls the contraction and expansion of the crystalline lens.

The third, inner layer or retina is a continuation of the optic nerve—located in the rear of the eye—a direct outgrowth of the brain. The retina is extremely thin and fine, and images of the outer world are cast upon it. Eyesight cannot function without the retina.

The Eye's "Yellow Spot": Secret to Vision

The macula or "yellow spot" is a part of the retina that allows details to enter into our vision. The center of the yellow spot is called the fovea centralis. This central pit sees twice as well as the retina itself, particularly in bright light. When you gaze at an object or point, the central pit sees the central area of focus and objects around that point are seen with the rest of the macula. By focusing on an object or letter for a second or two, the fovea enables you see twice as well as otherwise.

How the Eyes "See"

Eyesight consists of more than the eyeball itself. It is connected to the optical apparatus, buried deep in the socket and connected to the brain itself. Rays of light converge upon the retina and form an inverted image, which is transmitted by the optic nerve to the brain, which gives us vision. Light rays reflected from an object of vision focus directly on the retina. However, if the eyeball is too short from front to back, light rays coming in will not focus when they hit the retina—they will diffuse or spread out, causing blurred vision. This happens because the retina is stimulated in too many places instead of at a single point. This is called farsightedness. In nearsightedness, the eyeball becomes elongated so that the light rays entering it are focused before they reach the retina.

EYE MUSCLE ACCOMMODATION: MYSTERY UNVEILED

In order to "see" properly, the eyes must accommodate. Accommodation takes place when focusing on various distances—close and far. While looking at an object more than twenty feet away, light rays come into the eyes parallel. When looking at a close point, the rays come into the eyes at an angle. The eyes must accommodate these rays by adjusting the shape of the eye so that the rays will focus on the retina. This is accomplished by lengthening the eyeball. There is disagreement among ophthalmologists about which muscles are doing the focusing during accommodation. Dr. Helmholtz, an early eye doctor, said that accommodation is due to the expansion and contraction of the crystalline lens, caused by the action of the ciliary muscle. The Helmholtz theory is the accepted belief of most modern eyeglass doctors.

However, Dr. William H. Bates, the famous natural eye specialist, felt that the oblique eye muscles (running front to back above and below the orb of the eye) perform eye accommodation by compressing the round eyeball in the middle and making it longer horizontally. Dr. Bates cut these muscles in rabbits and found the eyes could not accommodate. When he injected a drug to paralyze the oblique muscles, the eyes failed to accommodate. When he put together the severed muscles and washed out the drug, the rabbits' eyes were able to accommodate again. The experiments done by Dr. Bates prove that it is not the crystalline lens but the external muscles that act upon the eyeball to give the eye its ability to adjust. This is supported by the fact that patients who have had their crystalline lens removed are still able to see, and have the power to accommodate.

In fact, the ciliary muscles work in conjunction with the external (oblique and recti) muscles and the iris to enable the eyes to accommodate properly. When the normal eye is looking at a close object the oblique muscles lengthen the eyeball so the rays can focus easily on the macula. The recti and ciliary muscles shorten the eyeball when the eyes are focused upon a distant point. The iris adjusts the size of the pupil for the amount of light necessary to see clearly. In a healthy eye, the pupil is smaller when viewing a distant sight, and grows larger when seeing a close object. In dim light the iris opens the pupil so that more light is let in, while on a bright sunny day the iris closes the pupil to prevent glare. As you can readily see, the iris also helps to accommodate the rays of light, so that a clear focus can be registered on the macula.

In short, the external muscles focus the rays of light, the iris adjusts the light, and the ciliary muscle focuses on the object. It is a very simple but profound process.

What Causes Weak Eye Muscles?

Tests on thousands of people over the years have proven beyond doubt that in most cases weak vision is caused by strain on the eye muscles. Eyestrain causes tense eye muscles; as the tense muscles are connected to the eyeball, they eventually distort the shape of the eye. Myopia (nearsightedness) means that the eyeball is elongated; hypermetropia (farsightedness) and presbyopia (farsightedness occurring in middle and old age) mean that the eyeball is flattened. This is caused by defective accommodation, which is caused by weak, unbalanced eye muscles. A myopic eye is "frozen" in an elongated position, making it hard to see objects in the distance. The farsighted eye is "frozen" in a flat position, making it hard to see near objects. Thus a fundamental principle in eye improvement training is that relaxation of the tension in the eye muscles and strengthening of weak eye muscles can definitely make weak or defective eyes strong again.

How Good Is Your Peripheral Vision?

In the normal healthy eye peripheral vision is quite clear. Its range is very wide and high. However, peripheral vision is weakened by squinting, too much reading, heavy concentration, mental tension, and malnutrition. The first three causes tend to center attention on a point, while leaving out the side areas. Dr. Bates says, "The normal eye sees one thing *best*, but not one thing only." In chapter 4 we will discuss a peripheral vision technique to improve your side vision.

GAINING HEALTHY VIBRANT EYES

The eyes cannot be treated as an unconnected isolated organ. There is an intimate association between the liver, blood, nervous system, and eyes. When the body cells and liver become weak, toxic, and unhealthy, the eyes reflect this weakened condition. If the colon is toxic and blocked with wastes, the blood becomes impure, health declines, and the eyes will become weak and drab, with heavy dark circles around them. On the other hand, a clean blood stream and a healthy functioning liver heal and strengthen the eyes.

Do you want healthy vibrant eyes? Then you must build up your health and vitality through diet, exercise, and eye training methods. Of prime importance is wholesome, unprocessed foods and thorough bowel elimination, two to three times a day.

Are Eyeglasses or Contacts Necessary?

Eyeglasses and contact lenses are at best a "crutch" for the eyes; they do not halt poor vision or stop the cause of faulty vision. And, in fact, full strength glasses "fix" the eyes in a permanently locked position, which prevents the eye muscles from focusing on near or far objects. Strong glasses with thick lenses always weaken the eyes. We need to look for and correct the individual cause or causes of weak vision, which are usually poor eye habits, poor nutrition, excessive eyestrain, close work, and so on.

However, that doesn't mean you should make the mistake I (Mantak Chia) made when I first started natural eye training. I threw away my eyeglasses. But striving to see without glasses too soon places excess strain and tension on the eyes and brain. So discarding my glasses while my eyes were still weak actually slowed down my eye improvement for many years. Please learn from my personal experience and continue to wear glasses while you undertake this program, especially if your vision is very weak and blurry.

Instead of abruptly stopping to use your glasses, you can begin with removing your glasses at odd times during the day to accustom your eyes to seeing naturally without them. You can also visit your local optometrist and ask for weaker lenses, or ask that your present glasses be ground down half a diaptor. Vision therapists often prescribe a 20–30 lens as a beginning point. Then, as your vision fitness improves over time, order weaker lenses for your glasses until you reach a point where they can be dispensed with entirely. Do not rush this process. Take enough time to strengthen your eyes with these powerful eye-training methods before you discontinue using glasses.

When your vision reaches 20–50 without glasses, you can take your glasses off without undue strain. Of course, you may still need to wear glasses while driving or looking into the distance. Once you are able to see 20–30 or better, you can dispense with glasses entirely. If you have close vision problems (farsightedness), wear the weakest lens that still enables you to see the print. Gradually have the lens weakened until you no longer need glasses to perform close work or reading.

How Long Does It Take to Achieve 20–20 Vision?

Working with natural eye training methods takes time. Just how long it takes varies from person to person, as everyone has different eye conditions. It all depends on how poor your vision is and how long you have worn glasses or contacts. However, if you thoroughly understand and apply these natural eye teachings, your vision will improve at a faster pace.

If your vision is 20–50 or less, it may take a few weeks to a few months to bring your vision back to normal (20–20). If you have

20–70 to 20–100 vision, it may take several months to a year. If you have 20–200 or worse, it may take a few years. It all depends on your understanding, dedication, and consistent practice of these special eye-training techniques. You are the only one who can improve your vision. Stick to it! You must give it time.

Seventy-five percent of Americans are vision impaired! How would you like to be among the 25 percent with strong sharp vision? If you follow the eye instructions in this book faithfully and persistently, you too may soon have perfect sight without glasses.

No matter how long it takes, the goal is to become naturally visually fit. Most people after the age of forty-five require glasses and begin losing their vision. You will not lose your vision, even into advanced age, if you perform these exercises conscientiously. If you consult with a natural vision instructor your eyesight will improve faster, because a person with that expertise can show you how to relax your mind, body, and eyes.

Knowledge and Wisdom Bring Understanding and Practice

When you understand how the eye functions, you will practice the eye exercises with knowledge and insight. The eye is an intricate organ of the body, connected to the brain, nervous system, and bloodstream, and can be strengthened and rejuvenated just as any other muscle or organ of the body. Eyesight is a marvelous miracle of creation. If the eyes are not abused they will take care of you for a long, healthy, and happy life.

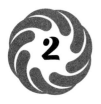

The Basic Foundation of Eye Improvement

FOUR EXTRAORDINARY TEN-MINUTE EYE IMPROVEMENT TECHNIQUES

These four amazing ten-minute eye improvement techniques developed by Dr. William Bates and Margaret Corbett—Sunning, Palming, the Long Swing, and Black Period Eye Gazing—are key to better vision. Dr. Bates based his methods on the principle of relaxation. Margaret Corbett wrote two eye books, *How to Improve Your Eyes* in 1938 and *Help Yourself to Better Sight* in 1949.

Margaret Corbett also organized a school of visual education in Los Angeles, California, for students and teachers. Many of the teachers she instructed are still teaching today throughout the world. I (Mantak Chia) was instructed in natural eye training for three years by Helen Tolmich, who was a student teacher under Margaret Corbett. Margaret Corbett's eyesight was so clear that—even when she was past ninety years of age—she could see the stars during daylight hours.

During the odd moments of the day, practice this short program of four ten-minute techniques. They are the cornerstone of your eye improvement practice. When you learn to totally relax with these four exceptional mind-eye-body relaxation exercises, you will see dramatic improvement in your vision. Be consistent with these techniques and you'll be delighted with the results!

Eye Technique Number 1: Sunning

Without the sun, the earth and all life on it would cease to exist. The eyes function only in light. The lack of light can seriously impact eye health: coal miners have observed that mules kept in a dark coal mine eventually lose their sight. Many nervous people dread the sunlight, and unwittingly cover their eyes with dark sunglasses. But wearing dark shades does not overcome the fear of sunlight (photophobia) or improve vision. The constant use of sunglasses and hanging out in dark places make the eyes dull and unable to take even the smallest amount of sunlight or brightness.

Photophobia can only be cured by light itself, eye exercises, and good dietary habits. Light sensitivity can be easily overcome by practicing the Sunning technique. The sun improves the eyes and pupils in many wonderful ways. For instance, it loosens tight muscles. The nerves and muscles just naturally let go of stress and tension, a leading cause of weakened eyesight. Well-sunned eyes sparkle and retain their beauty and luster. If you want shining, magnetic eyes, give up the habit of wearing sunglasses. They deprive the eyes of needed light, weaken eye function, and can lead to blindness! The eyes require outdoor light—give plenty of it to them.

Performing the Sunning Eye Technique

The Sunning technique is an excellent exercise for relaxing the eyes and helping to overcome the fear of light. "Sun" your eyes regularly in the following manner:

1. Sit down, relax your mind and body, and loosen your neck and shoulders.
2. Next, close your eyes and swing your head side to side easily while

facing the sun. (On sunless days, use a 150- or 250-watt reflector spotlight bulb. Sit 6 feet away from the bulb.) Turn your head gently toward your left shoulder, then swing it back easily to your right shoulder. Continue this movement for 5 minutes and enjoy the warm feeling of the sun bathing your eyes. You will soon feel a sense of peace and relaxation.

With practice, you will start to notice an "optical illusion"—the sun itself will seem to move to the right as you swing your head to the left and vice versa. Remember to keep your eyes closed throughout the exercise.

The sun is a wonderful eye restorer. Make use of this heaven-sent miracle, and experience the miracle of perfect eyesight in your life. After you finish Sunning, perform eye technique number two, Palming. The sun feeds the nerves, brain, and muscles of the eyes and Palming creates darkness, allowing the eye to *rest*.

Are Sunglasses Harmful?

Millions of sunglasses are sold year round, throughout the world, with no consideration given to their damaging effect upon the eyes. Sunglasses shield our eyes from the life-giving sun. Some eye specialists warn against the excessive use of sunglasses. They are frustrated by their inability to do anything about this worldwide sunglass epidemic. The bad habit of wearing dark sunglasses makes the pupil stay in an enlarged position. Continued use of eyeshades over time actually paralyzes the pupil of the eye. Living indoors all day long does the same thing.

In bright light the pupil becomes smaller and in darkness it becomes larger. Wearing sunglasses in sunlight keeps the pupil expanded because the shaded lens does not allow light to enter. When the pupil is stuck in this enlarged position, the bright daylight seems even brighter. This is what weakens our eyes. If you are driving into the sunset or sunrise, use your sunglasses to reduce glare;

otherwise, leave them off. You can also purchase Dr. Ott's full spectrum sunglasses. They take out the sun glare and let in beneficial light rays.

If the sun bothers your eyes, the best remedy is to spend more time outdoors in the daylight and secondly, consume a better diet, consisting of whole grains, vegetables, fruits, seeds, and protein for your individual body type (see chapter 8). Two of the greatest foods for the eyes are sunflower seeds and parsley. They contain vitamin B_2, which helps to overcome light sensitivity. If you avoid the sun completely, you'll become oversensitive to even ten minutes of it. Get some sun, within reason.

Eye Technique Number 2: The Palming Technique

Palming—cupping your closed eyes with your palms—is one of the most important methods for relaxing eye muscles and nerves. When performed regularly, this superior technique can bring about a complete transformation and restoration of your eyes. Palming helps to calm the mind, improve color clarity, and to prevent many degenerative eye conditions. Palming is practiced and taught by many visual training teachers, naturopaths, and holistic doctors throughout the world, as well as by the yogis of India, Chinese Taoists, and Tibetan monks.

When you first start Palming, you may see gray or white light or colors. As you continue practicing, however, you will see only black darkness. You will reach a state of calm, with your mind relaxed, which will enable your eyes to heal and regenerate quickly.

When Palming, do not place undue pressure on your face. Any pressure on the lids or face interferes with nerve and blood circulation to the eyes. You want free circulation to your eyes at all times. Also, make sure you can breathe easily and deeply through your nose. Inhale, exhale, relax, and let go of tension in the eyes, face, forehead, jaws, teeth, and neck.

Performing the Palming Technique

Perform the Palming technique for 5 to 10 minutes with your elbows on your thighs or on a table. You can also place a cushion under your elbows for both positions.

1. Place your cupped palms over your closed eyelids without touching them.
2. Next, imagine something pleasant and let blackness come into your field of vision. If you see lights and colors, you are not totally relaxed—it's a sign of anxiety and mental activity. You will be relaxed when you can experience and see total blackness while Palming. Blackness equals healing, rest, and relaxation for the eyes. The positive benefit is improved vision, clarity of mind, and sharp-focusing eye muscles.

Eye Technique Number 3: The Long Swing Technique

The natural holistic health view of disease says: "There is but one disease, toxemia or congestion; there is but one cure, good circulation." Wherever there is a blockage or congestion in the body, energy and healing cannot take place. We need to unblock the blockage, then energy and healing flow with ease. Relaxing the body also relaxes the mind and eyes, while a tense body causes tension in both. Illness, toxemia, poor digestion, and a toxic, congested colon are prime causes of eye problems.

Dr. Bates and Margaret Corbett emphasized the fact that tension causes congestion—its cure is relaxation, permitting circulation to flow naturally. Deep relaxation is also the secret of the Taoist Chi Kung exercise movements. Taoist masters teach us to attain deep relaxation while performing the exercises, thereby allowing a great surge and inflow of chi (spiritual and physical healing energy) to circulate throughout the body. With healing chi energy flowing smoothly in the body, we can enjoy super health and a tranquil mind.

There are two types of relaxation. One is the "rag doll" limp or passive relaxation; the other is known as dynamic relaxation—exercising, working, and moving about while being relaxed.

The Long Swing technique, sometimes called the Elephant Swing, was practiced and taught by the Taoist Chi Kung schools in China for centuries. Dr. Bates discovered the Long Swing in the early 1900s. He discovered that when the Long Swing is performed correctly, the eyesight improved more quickly than with any other method he taught. It is a dynamic relaxation technique.

In most physical exercises from the West (weightlifting, weight machines, calisthenics, and so on), the muscles become tense or tighten up. This tightness is the opposite of relaxation. Chi Kung movements like the Long Swing are performed in a relaxed manner for maximum benefit. If you do perform weight resistance exercises, never strain or force the weight to move. Exercise without strain, and your muscles will build up naturally, almost without effort. Always finish off your resistance exercise routine with yoga, stretching, the Long Swing, and other loosening Chi Kung exercises. Then you will have the best of both worlds—yang or hard toning exercises and yin or soft relaxation exercises. You'll see great improvement in your vision if you follow such a program.

How does one relax? First loosen the nerves and muscles, then relax the mind. Shake your arms and legs, roll your neck, relax your jaw, then empty your mind—just put your attention on your movement and breathing. Swinging is one of the easiest ways to relax the mind, body, and spirit. Children swing and move their bodies in all different ways. They are happy and have not a care in the world. They are relaxed and flexible—nothing bothers them for very long. We need to become like little children in this respect and not be so uptight and hard in our attitudes.

The Long Swing helps to release the energy in the nerves and muscles; it loosens every vertebra in the spinal column and relaxes the internal organs, thus improving the eyesight, as well as the general health and energy of the body.

Performing the Long Swing

1. Stand with your feet parallel, about 10 inches apart.
2. Shift your weight from one foot to the other, by lifting the heel of each foot as you turn in a swaying motion (fig. 2.1). As you sway gently from one side to the other, turn your head and shoulders while swinging, and let your arms hang loosely—let them swing freely as you turn. Move as if you are dancing! Move with an easy rhythm. Always remember that your head moves with your body, not by itself.

   Your chest, shoulders, face, legs, and neck must be soft and relaxed. Count each swing aloud; this stops you from holding your breath. Never hold your breath during relaxation exercises. Easy relaxed breathing is necessary to let go of body tension and mental stress.

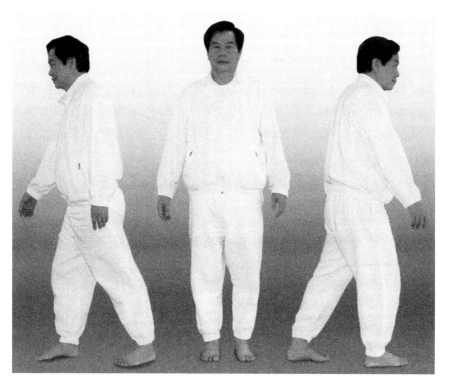

Fig. 2.1. The Long Swing Technique

Notice the room "moving" past you in the opposite direction. When you notice this illusion, the eyes will begin to shift naturally. Let your eyes allow the room to pass by without becoming fixed on anything. Let the room swing by, or as Dr. Bates said, "Let the world go by." Keep your mind on the illusion of the "moving room." The swinging illusion tricks the eyes to loosen and relax, and also breaks the fixed-eye staring habit. It will allow the eyes to shift 70 times per second, a natural occurrence in good healthy eyesight. *Swing, relax, and see!* Perform 60 to 100 swinging movements, 1 or 2 sessions a day.

Practice the Long Swing for a few minutes before going to bed, upon arising, or after Palming. Dr. Bates says: "The Long Swing relieves pain, fatigue, dizziness, and other symptoms because the swing brings about relief from the effort of trying to see." It relaxes the entire body-mind-eye complex.

Eye Technique Number 4: The Black Period Eye-Gazing Technique

The Black Period technique has been used for years in the Dr. Bates' eye training system. We feel that it is a premier technique to sharpen both close and distant vision.

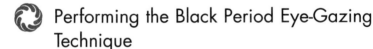 ## Performing the Black Period Eye-Gazing Technique

When performing this technique, practice first with one eye at a time (cover one eye with an eye patch or your hand), then use both eyes together. Remember to close your eyes for 10 seconds after each Black Period Gazing session.

1. From the text of a book, pick out a period that you can see clearly and sharply from a distance. Make sure you have lots of light shining on the page. To improve close vision (farsightedness), place the

period 10 inches or less away from your eyes. To improve distance vision (nearsightedness), place the period 2 feet or more away from your eyes. Gazing at the smallest period you can see will sharpen your vision more quickly!

2. Gaze at the period for 15 seconds—look inside the period and trace the edge of it with your eyes. Relax your eyes and gaze lightly at the period.

This Black Period Eye-Gazing technique can be done any time during the day or during your eye training sessions. It is an excellent exercise for keeping good vision, because it enables the eyes to focus directly on the macula—the center of eyesight.

THREE MASTER FORMULAS FOR PERFECT EYESIGHT

It has been discovered in ancient writings from ages past that the brain/mind and the eyes operate in close harmony. Defective eyesight can be improved by mental methods accompanied by proper eye habits, eye exercises, diet, and physical relaxation techniques.

Three amazing formulas are derived from the knowledge that the secret to perfect eyesight lies in the coordination between the brain and the muscles controlling the movements of the eyeball.

Master Eye Formula Number 1: Relax the Eye Muscles

Abnormal strain of the external muscles of the eyes is always associated with a strained, unnatural effort to see. When this strain is stopped, the eye muscles become normal and all errors of refraction vanish like magic. A different kind of strain results in each error of refraction (such as nearsightedness, farsightedness, and so on). Relaxing any type of eyestrain will relieve that particular error of refraction, and total relaxation of eye, mind, and body will reduce them all.

Master Eye Formula Number 2:
Relax the Brain and Mind

The strain of your eyes to see is literally a strain of your mind; conversely, when your mind strains, it is reflected as a strain of the eyes. There is thus a very true connection between stressed-out mental states and defective eyesight; they each act upon and react to the other in a cause-and-effect relationship.

Dr. Bates once said:

> When the mind is at rest, nothing can tire the eyes; and when the mind is under a strain nothing can rest them; anything that rests the mind will benefit the eyes.

Master Eye Formula Number 3:
Reduce Mental Strain and Strengthen Eye Muscles

The only real treatment for regaining your lost eyesight begins by relieving mental stress and physical strain, followed by a recovery of the mental control of the eye muscles. The vision exercises in this book will help you to reduce strain and allow your eye muscles to strengthen and function in a relaxed manner, as they were meant to do.

Do you want perfect eyesight? Develop mental poise and balance—a prerequisite of mental relaxation and removal of strain. Learn to let go of mental strain, worry, fear, anxiety, and so on. Practice mental calm and watch your eyesight improve by quantum leaps.

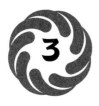

Daily Eye-Strengthening Habits

FOURTEEN HABITS FOR HEALTHY VISION

In this chapter we will discuss fourteen daily eye-strengthening habits and the reasons for them. These habits can be easily adopted and most can be performed throughout the day, such as while you are waiting in line at the store, driving, stopped in traffic, or even while reading, watching television, walking, and so on. They are enjoyable to do, and will extend your clear vision well into advanced age.

Eye Habit Number 1: Relax Your Eyes

Myopia (nearsightedness) has two causes:

1. Not focusing or using the eyes enough while looking into the distance
2. Performing excessive close work

Unfortunately, we live in a close-vision world. Reading (books, magazines, and newspapers) and precision work in our offices, factories, and schools all require extreme close vision for hours at a time. In addition, twenty-first-century life has reduced the need for clear, distance eyesight. Many people rarely look at an object more than fifty feet away. This has caused an epidemic of weak distant vision.

Gazing into the distance (twenty or more feet away) is the natural position of the eye. Ciliary eye muscles *relax* when viewing objects more than twenty feet away because the rays of light come in parallel. During close work, light flows into the eyes diversely; the ciliary muscles have to contract to properly focus the light upon the macula. When these muscles are kept in constant contraction for long periods, they tend to remain cramped. Then, when you look up, the vision becomes fuzzy. This is similar to what happens when you hold a barbell in a fully flexed arm curl position for several minutes: your biceps and fingers cramp tight. When the weight is put down, your fingers take a minute to "uncurl" themselves from their contracted grip on the bar. The biceps also remains tight and contracted momentarily. In the same way, too much close work cramps the eye muscles in one position.

Most of us start out in life with good vision, but after high school and college and years in front of a computer, we end-up with "thick-window-pane glasses." Our health and vision deteriorate in spite of our material knowledge and credentials. We need wisdom with knowledge to give us true understanding of how the eyes function and how to improve our vision.

Relax Your Eyes—Part I: Practice distance seeing

Do you want clear, sharp vision? Then you must practice distance seeing. Practice distance gazing while walking or during lunch breaks—look out the window into the distance to distinguish objects at or slightly beyond the far limits of what you can see now. Focus on objects you can see clearly and strive to bring them into clearer focus for a few seconds; this will help you to regain distance vision if it is weak or blurry.

Practice looking at things in an effortless and relaxed manner.

Never strain. It is important that you not gaze at objects you cannot see well—this strains the eyes even more! Read distant signs, distinguish license plate numbers of passing cars. Watch birds in flight. Look at distant airplanes. Count stars at night.

Relax Your Eyes—Part II: Look up from your close work

This is an important eye habit you can practice while reading, at work, or watching television. It helps to prevent the eyes from getting into a frozen position.

Simply look *up* from your close work every five minutes and gaze at a distant object for five seconds. Drs. Ross and Rehner, natural eye doctors, advise: "Look up and away from your close work at frequent intervals. No matter how fascinating or important your reading, drawing, or sewing may be, glance away from it for a few seconds every five minutes." They suggest that this simple habit be continued even when your sight has returned to normal.

Relax Your Eyes—Part III: Avoid close work during and after meals

Dr. Sasaki, a Japanese eyesight specialist, states that you can add twenty years to your life if you do not read while eating, and go outdoors after meals for at least thirty to sixty minutes. Reading and close work during and after meals impair the eyesight because digestion draws blood to the digestive system, thus causing lack of nutrients to the eyes, weak eye muscles, and cloudy vision.

Going outside after meals provides the necessary oxygen to properly digest and assimilate food. Spending an hour outdoors after meals vastly enhances digestive powers, which improves and strengthens eyesight. Humans require large amounts of outdoor oxygen, especially for the kidneys, liver, and eyes. This imparts vigorous health and superior eyesight. Breathing in outdoor oxygen and performing deep breathing exercises in the fresh outdoor air helps in the production of healthy red blood cells; it improves cellular oxygen; and it gives us inspiration, good health, and long life. Take advantage of the outdoors often, especially in warm, sunny weather.

Important Eye Note: Myopics (nearsighted people) attempt to see a whole object, such as a car or building, at once. Those with poor close vision (farsighted) attempt to see a whole page. Keep in mind that the eyes can only see one part best for clear sharp vision.

Eye Habit Number 2: Avoid Strain

Strain is the major cause of imperfect eyesight. Straining to see any object, far or near, which you are unable to see clearly, places a heavy strain on the eye muscles. Just as straining to lift a heavy weight can strain a tendon or muscle, straining to read fine print in poor lighting causes weak vision at the close point (farsightedness). Holding the print too close (less than twelve inches), reading excessively, and straining to "make out" objects in the distance are the major causes of nearsightedness (myopia).

The correct method to avoid strain is to: 1) read in good bright light; 2) while reading or performing close work, focus in on a letter on the page every few minutes, and gaze at it for five to ten seconds. If you cannot see an object clearly, do not strain to see it. Instead, you should move closer to the object, use brighter lighting, or temporarily wear glasses.

Eyestrain is also caused by long exposure to cold wind in the eyes and bright artificial lights (especially fluorescent lights). Excessive watching of television or movies strains tired weak eyes. To strengthen, heal, and relax your tired and strained eyes, look at nature's outdoor bounties: green trees, green grass, mountains, beautiful flowers, flowing rivers, blue-green oceans, the open sky, the stars at night, the moon, the sun at sunrise or sunset—nature herself. She is the only one who can heal you, with the help of healing chi energy from the heavens.

Avoid Strain—Part I: Do not read when tired or sick

The body is a flowing, dynamic energy machine. When the body is ill or tired, the eyes also become tired and blurry. Weak bodily energy weakens the entire system, especially the liver, which is directly connected to the eyes via the acupuncture meridians. Reading during illness or fatigue weakens the focusing eye muscles.

Do you remember a past illness or stress situation you had? You can bet your eyesight became dim or cloudy during that period. In my teens I (Mantak Chia) did plenty of reading late at night when I could scarcely keep my eyes open; this was a great strain on my eyes. Consequently, my eyesight weakened. The rule of thumb here is to read or perform close work when your energy is high; during illness or fatigue obtain plenty of rest and sleep.

Important Note: The body, mind, and eyes heal and rejuvenate during rest and a good solid night's sleep. Lack of sufficient rest and sleep can easily run down your immune system, liver, and gastrointestinal system, and result in poor vision.

Avoid Strain—Part II: Refrain from reading in poor lighting

Nature, or outside solar light, gives us 10,000 watts of bright light. Inside lighting is very dim in comparison, seldom reaching 150–200 watts. Most people read with 60–100 watt bulbs or less and strain their eyes. If you have trouble reading in dim light, your eyes will strain and weaken even more.

It is best to read in daylight, with the sun or outdoor light coming through the window onto your reading or working material. Or better yet, do your reading or close work outdoors when the weather is clear and pleasant. When night approaches, make sure you shine a bright bulb—150–200 watts—onto your reading material to make it clear and to lessen eyestrain. Adjust the light so it does not cause a glare on the page. Dr. Vogel recommends against reading at night before bed or in bed, as this can further weaken vision, and cause bloodshot eyes, fatigue, and insomnia.

Avoid Strain—Part III: Maintain a good posture while reading

Poor posture while reading is a major cause of weakened and fatigued eyesight. Avoid slumping or hanging or craning your head down while reading. Sit comfortably erect. A slumped head position causes the eyes to point downward. This causes gravity to pull down on the eyeballs, which places strain on the extrinsic eye muscles, which hold the eyes back in the sockets. Holding this "neck bent downward" position causes lengthening of the eyeball, resulting in myopia or nearsightedness.

Avoid Strain—Part IV: Hold print parallel twenty inches from the eyes

Many myopics can improve their sight by adopting this one important eye habit of holding print parallel twenty inches from the eyes. Holding the print too close to the eyes is a major cause of myopia. When I observe young people holding their reading material too close to their eyes (less than twelve inches), I know they are heading for myopic vision. Dr. Sasaki and many other natural eye doctors do not recommend excessive reading for youngsters; they suggest instead that youngsters read only when necessary and gaze into the distance as often a possible.

Avoid Strain—Part V: Avoid reading more than thirty minutes at a time

Thirty minutes is about the maximum time the eyes can handle without strain or fatigue. Read for a while, then get up and walk around, stretch or go outside for a breath of fresh air. Look into the distance. Take a deep breath, bend over and rub your face, forehead, and around the eyes, exhale and stand straight. Inhale again and bend backward, then to each side, and exhale and relax your gaze. Then do the Palming method taught by Dr. Bates: close your eyes and place your palms over your eye sockets and visualize something very black, such as black velvet.

Deep breathing, face and head rubbing, bending and twisting, and Palming all help to refresh the brain and eyes, imparting increased energy and clear thinking. Make it your refreshment break instead of coffee or soda.

Eye Habit Number 3: Invigorating Lemon Juice Eye Bath

Dr. William Apt, a leading eye specialist in the mid-1900s, recommended the Lemon Juice Eye Bath. He learned this secret from a 105-year-old man who instructed Dr. Apt to "put three or four drops of lemon juice in an eyecup with purified water and wash each eye with it daily for about 20–30 seconds." Dr. Apt says it is invigorating and strengthening. It removes toxic fatigue of the eye. The ancient oldster who taught Dr. Apt washes his eyes daily, eats natural foods, wears no glasses, and has perfect eyesight! The Lemon Juice Eye Bath is also recommended as a cure for cataracts, when used along with osteopathic treatment, plus a strict seven-day elimination (vegetable and fruit) diet, once a month.

Eye Habit Number 4: Healing Sun

Healing Sun—Part I: Sunshine is food for the eyes

Sunlight is "food" for the eyes. They are nourished and healed by its warm radiating energy. Humans thrive on outdoor oxygen and sunlight. We live on a carbon-based planet, filled with oxygen and solar light. The human body was designed by nature to be an outdoor dweller most of the time. This is our human biological destiny.

We have switched our position in the scheme of things and fallen prey to our own arrogance and ignorance. Now we suffer from lack of sun and air, while nature is there waiting for us to partake of her fragrance, beauty, and bounty. One of the major causes of poor eyesight in this so-called "modern society" is staying indoors during daylight hours.

Go outdoors in the sunlight every day—walk when you can, work in the garden, read a book, gaze into the distance, enjoy sports. Whatever you enjoy, do more of it in the life-giving sun and fresh air. Well-sunned eyes glow with magnetism and health. Outdoor people generally have better vision than indoor dwellers. The famous old-time lion tamer Johnny Pack enjoyed several hours a day of sunshine. At ninety-one years young in 1996, he had excellent eyesight at both far and close point.

The best time to enjoy the sunshine is in the morning before 11:00 a.m. or after 3:00 p.m. The sun produces 10,000 watts of natural light; indoor bulbs are a weak 100 watts in comparison. On hot days, walk in the shade and gaze into the distance. You will soon adjust to the light and even enjoy it.

Healing Sun—Part II: Perform Yoga Sun Gazing

How would you like to possess magnetic healthy eyes? Develop a steady powerful gaze? Approach life situations without fear? The ancient yogis use this as a meditation technique to infuse the body, mind, and spirit with light and power.

Performing the Yoga Sun Gazing Exercise

1. Go outside at sunrise or sunset when the orb is red or orange. Open your eyes wide and take in 9 deep breaths (in and out gently) while looking at the sun. Feel the "sun energy" traveling into your eyes and down to your bellybutton area (*hara*).

2. After sun gazing, gently cover your eyes with your palms for a few minutes while visualizing the color black. This helps to relax and heal stress and tension in the mind and eyes.

Being exposed to plenty of sunshine, allowing fresh air to hit your bare skin, and walking on the earth with bare feet all help to improve eyesight. Practice these golden treasures whenever possible. The immortal Taoist masters cherish these activities, along with Chi Kung exercises, as the keys to health, energy, and longevity.

Eye Habit Number 5: Oriental Yang Eye Candle Gazing Technique

This powerful Yang Eye Candle Gazing technique has been taught and practiced in the East for thousands of years. It is known to result in glowing magnetic eyes that can look anyone in the eye without fear or timidity.

This technique not only improves the eyesight, but was known by the ancient Taoist masters to alleviate many eye problems and latent ailments within the body. The whites of the eyes will become clear and your eyes will shine with brightness.

Performing the Yang Eye Candle Gazing Technique

1. Light a candle and sit in front of it at arm's length and at eye level. Gaze steadily at it without blinking.
2. Breathe naturally, and continue gazing for 5 minutes without moving your body. Try not to move your eyelids. Less movement brings more magnetic power and control into the eyes and nervous system.
3. Keep your eyes open and allow the tears to flow down your cheeks; open your eyes wider as the tears flow down.
4. Every minute or so, close your eyes for 10 or 15 seconds.
5. Finish by closing your eyes and Palming for 2 minutes to cool down your eyes.

Eye Habit Number 6:
Indian Yoga Nasal Massage Technique

Indian ayurvedic medicine teaches us that chronic colds, flu, mucus, and lung congestion are the basic causes of most eye problems, as the eyes are in close proximity to the nasal and sinus passages.

Nasal massage helps to improve sinus conditions and allows you to see objects with clarity. It also helps to relieve emotional tension, which builds up in the face, forehead, and eyes when we are under stress.

Performing the Yoga Nasal Massage Technique

Dip your little finger into sesame oil or one drop of eucalyptus or lavender oil. Insert it into each nostril and slowly massage as deeply as possible in a clockwise and then counterclockwise direction. Gently massage the inside nose tissue each morning before breakfast at least 3 times a week.

You may feel soreness. Go easy. You may also sneeze and blow your nose several times. Don't panic. This is a "cleansing action" taken by your body. It'll clear your sinuses pronto! This massage opens up the breathing channels, releases pent-up emotions, and improves eye clarity.

Eye Habit Number 7:
Taoist Kidney, Stomach, and Liver Massage—
Key to Super Health and Clear Vision

In addition to the essential role that the kidneys, stomach, and liver play in the health of the whole body, these organs are respectively linked to the ears, mouth, and eyes. When they are healthy, the eyes are too. In Chinese medicine, the kidneys are considered the health and longevity organs of the body. Weaken the kidneys and the health of the entire body begins to fail. The stomach is considered the central energy station or grand central station for food distribution to the entire system. The liver is the great detoxifying organ of the body. It filters out chemicals, pollutants, preservatives, fats, oils, and so on. A weak liver places great stress on the immune system. Congestion in the liver causes poor food digestion and fatigue; it can easily lead to yeast infections, PMS, and blood disorders.

These internal organ massage techniques, performed regularly, can help improve vision and increase overall health.

Performing the Kidney Massage

1. Rub your hands together until hot and place them over the kidneys (right and left side of lower back) for 10 seconds.
2. Vigorously rub the kidney area up and down at least 35 times.
3. Finish by lightly pounding the kidney area with your palms.

Performing the Stomach and Liver Massage

The liver is under the right rib cage. The stomach is under the left rib cage. This massage can help sharpen your vision and bring energy and healing power into your stomach and liver. Vigorously rub under the right and left sides of your rib cage 35 times each.

Eye Habit Number 8: Eye Massage with Palming

Acupressure has been around for thousands of years, and has more recently been introduced to the West by Chinese acupuncture masters. Acupressure is finger pressure therapy on meridian points or pathways that run up and down the body, arms, legs, head, and face.

Performing the Acupressure Eye Massage with Palming

1. Exert heavy finger pressure upon each of the points surrounding the eyes for 10 seconds (fig. 3.1).
2. Then rub each point for 5 seconds. Any pain denotes eye weakness. Healthy eyes have no pain, even under heavy finger pressure. If your eyes are very weak, spend more time on eye massage.
3. Next, with the pads of the first three fingertips, press lightly upon closed eyelids for 30 seconds—this helps myopia (nearsightedness).
4. Locate the *hoku* point on each hand (on the top of the hand, on the web where the thumb and the index finger meet) and massage for 30 seconds each (fig. 3.2).
5. Finish with Palming (fig. 3.3). Rub hands together until hot and place cupped palms over closed eyes for 30 seconds. Visualize dark black velvet; it is restful and healing for the eyes, mind, and entire body.

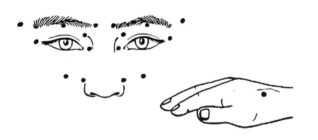 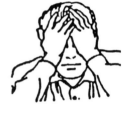

Fig. 3.1. Acupressure points around the eyes

Fig. 3.2. The hoku point on the hand

Fig. 3.3. Palming

Eye Habit Number 9:
Loosening Your Neck to Reduce Eye Tension

Tenseness around the neck and shoulders can cause severe eye tension. To loosen up your neck and release tension, do the following neck-loosening exercises. If you do these exercises several times a day, they will help to reduce eyestrain, neck tightness, and eye tension headaches.

 ## Powerful Neck-Loosening Exercises

1. Perform neck rolls, turning your head in a circular motion (fig. 3.4).
2. Move your head left to right as far as you can.
3. Let it drop forward and then backward as far as possible.
4. While your head is all the way back, lift both shoulders up and near your earlobes and move your head right to left and left to right several times. This movement squeezes the tension right out of the neck and trapezius muscles. You will feel relaxed and refreshed after performing this movement for 1 to 2 minutes.

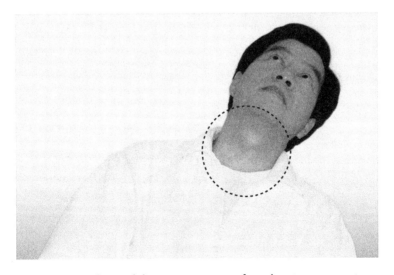

Fig. 3.4. Circular neck-loosening exercise for releasing eye tension

Eye Habit Number 10:
Taoist Do-In Eye Massage Techniques

Oriental Taoist and Zen masters practice a form of self-healing massage called Do-In. Do-In is a chi (energy) technique; it combines with Chi Kung breathing movements to revive and regenerate the body, mind, emotions, and spirit, harmonizing all levels of being with the rhythm of life. Practiced daily, Do-In will help you to maintain balance and harmony in life, to remain centered, grounded, and focused.

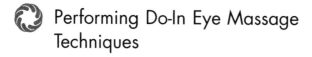 Performing Do-In Eye Massage Techniques

Massage Technique 1:
Scalp Rubbing Technique

Sit straight and relax mind and body. Simply rub your scalp with fingers slowly from front to back and in small circles for 30 to 60 seconds (fig. 3.5). This helps to clear the heart of toxins, relax the brain, calm nerves, invigorate the scalp, and improve eyesight by bringing blood circulation to the head and eye region. Even better, exchange scalp massages with your partner or friend. It's even more relaxing and soothing when someone else does it for you.

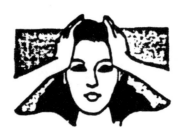

Fig. 3.5. Scalp massage reduces tension and stress.

❧ Massage Technique 2:
Palm Eye Massage Technique

1. Close eyes slightly and knead closed eyelids over eyeballs with the inside of your palms (fig. 3.6). Circle palms 16 times clockwise and 16 times counterclockwise.
2. Next, place palms on the eyes and move up and down 16 times, and side to side 16 times.

This is, from my (Mantak Chia) experience, the best eye massage to heal and prevent all conditions: nearsightedness, farsightedness, astigmatism, and the eye diseases of the middle-aged and elderly.

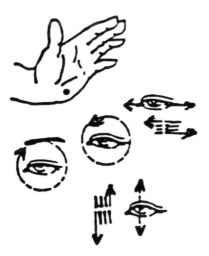

Fig. 3.6. Location of eye kneading

❧ Massage Technique 3:
Stroking Eyebrows Technique

Place thumbs on temple and stroke eyebrows with second knuckle of each forefinger, over eyebrows. Do this 16 times. Close the eyes and use light, even pressure. This helps to clear the eyes, regulate nerve function, and to prevent hardening of cerebral arteries and degenerative eye diseases.

❂ Massage Technique 4: Ironing the Face Technique

Scrub the face with open palms from the forehead down to the chin and then up to the ears in a circular motion, 16 times. The Chinese Taoists call this "Ironing the Face." It helps to remove wrinkles, brings fresh blood to the eyes, and improves the complexion.

Eye Habit Number 11: Squeeze Eyes Tightly and Open Eyes Widely

This Taoist eye technique increases circulation to the eyes, prevents watery eyes, and strengthens the eyelids and tear gland muscle (orbicularis palpebrarum), which normalizes the lachrymal glands. These glands furnish an alkaline solution that purifies the eyes and imparts a brilliant, sparkling luster to the eyes.

The healing sound sh-h-h-h-h-h-h is used to purify the liver and calm the nervous system (see chapter 5 for more on using this sound to heal the liver). Opening the eyes wide while exhaling the sound sh-h-h-h-h-h-h releases anger and tension from the liver and the eyes.

❂ Performing the Squeezing and Opening Eye Technique

1. Breathe in slowly and gradually squeeze your eyes tightly for 10 to 15 seconds.
2. Next, slowly exhale, making the sound sh-h-h-h-h-h-h while opening your eyes wide. Repeat 3–6 times.

Eye Habit Number 12: Naturopathic Eye Massage Technique

This eye massage technique was used by naturopathic doctors and health and physical culture practitioners in the 1800s to improve eyesight and prevent vision problems.

Performing the Naturopathic Eye Massage Technique

1. Place the palm of each hand on the bony ridge above each eye. Press hard on the brow and move the skin up and down, side to side, and in small circles. Perform each movement 12 times.

2. Place your open palms on each side of your temples. Move the skin up and down, forward and back, and in a circular motion. Perform each movement 12 times.

3. Place your fingers on each cheekbone under the eyes, then move the skin up and down, right and left. Perform each movement 12 times.

> *If you faithfully carry these instructions out it will prove*
> *of great importance in restoring your vision.*
>
> EDMUND SHAFTSBURY

Eye Habit Number 13: Tracking/Edging—Secret to Crystal Sharp Vision

How would you like to possess crystal sharp vision? Would you like to keep your vision when you are fifty, sixty, seventy, and beyond?

We are told that after forty years of age we will gradually lose the ability to focus at the close point, because the aging process produces a thickening in the lens of the eyes. Yet, myopics over the age of seventy can read fine print up close easily. How do the "experts" explain that? The truth is that the reason we lose our close vision and distant vision is because we have never learned, or we have forgotten, the habit of focusing. Dr. Bates called this "central fixation." When you lose the ability to focus, you tend to peer hard, staring fixedly and forcing yourself to see, or squinting your eyes. These bad eye habits will impair your eyes even further.

Our best vision comes when the rays of light focus directly into the macula area. A technique that modern pioneers in vision training refer to as "tracking" or "edging" helps to restore the natural ability to focus upon the macula. Tracking or edging is going around the outside perimeter of an object.

Performing the Tracking/Edging Eye Technique for Distant Vision

To improve your distant vision, track your eyes around a picture or a large letter on a sign that you can see clearly. Track around a table in the distance. Look up and down buildings, billboards, and highway signs. Edge along window frames, houses, and trees; use your imagination. At first, move slowly around the object, seeing each part of the edge. Later, as you become proficient, you can speed up the edging. As you practice objects will become sharp and clear to you. Practice outdoors! Sunlight makes everything clearer.

You can track by using your eyes only or you can use your nose as a focal point; this relaxes the head and neck, which prevents the eyes from staring with a fixed gaze. Point your nose at the object you have chosen and move the tip of the nose along its edges.

Remember to breathe deeply and easily while tracking. Tracking can be done anytime, such as while walking, looking out the window, reading, and so on. Close your eyes after tracking to rest them. Tracking can also be done with your eyes closed, by mentally remembering an object. If you are seeking super-sharp vision, practice tracking frequently.

Important Vision Training Note: Tracking is one of the most important eye improvement secrets I (Mantak Chia) have discovered in thirty years of research in my quest for perfect eyesight.

Performing the Tracking/Edging Eye Technique for Close Vision

1. To improve your close vision, track letters on the printed page: go around the outside and inside of the letter in all its details.
2. Each week, pick out smaller and smaller letters until you can read the smallest print easily.

Remember to close your eyes for a few moments between tracking sessions.

Eye Habit Number 14:
Head Lift Technique for Eye and Ear Problems

The Head Lift technique is an excellent result-producing exercise to clear up ear and eye problems. It also helps to overcome headaches and neck and shoulder pain.

 ## Performing the Head Lift Technique

1. Place both hands—fingers and palms—around the neck at the lower part of the skull (mastoid process).
2. Next, lift your head upward and a bit forward, while turning your head to the right as you are lifting.
3. Next, turn and lift head to the left in the same manner.

This simple movement can help unblock any pinched nerves in the neck or in the trapezius muscles, which are attached to the neck. Lift up your head gently, but do not squeeze the neck too hard. Turn as far as you can, comfortably, in each direction, without straining or jerking. Practice the Head Lift several times daily, especially before sleep.

Do-In Neck and Shoulder Massage

Along with the Head Lift technique, it is also a good idea to practice Do-In or Self-Massage to your neck and shoulders, with your fingers, knuckles, and palms. If you have any soreness or energy blockages in these areas, massaging them will help you to feel renewed energy and fresh blood flowing to your head, brain, and eyes. Without the proper nerve and blood supply to the eyes, vision improvement cannot progress at a steady rate. In fact, nerve and blood flow blockages can definitely hold back your quest for perfect eyesight. For faster eyesight improvement, the Head Lift technique is unsurpassed.

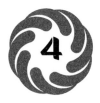

Perfect Eyesight Exercise Program

Eyes need exercise just as much as other muscles. If you were to place your arm in a brace for a few weeks it would start to get weaker and smaller because the blood would not be able to circulate sufficiently to impart strength and growth to the arm muscles. Similarly, when the muscles of the eye become weak, vision becomes unfocused and eyesight weakens. The eye muscles can lose their power to focus the eyeball on a close or distant point, resulting in nearsightedness or farsightedness.

Just as our arm muscles need exercise, our eyes also need to "pump iron." We can perform sets and reps of exercises to bring them back into focus. Eye muscles can be strengthened not only to correct problems but also to enhance vision, even to the point of being able to see telescopically. What others can see only with binoculars, a person with telescopic vision can see without them! Such super-vision is far above the average. But it can be achieved with work, persistence, and perseverance.

These exercises can also be fun and enjoyable if you do them with a happy, positive attitude. Take your time; no rushing; calm your mind; turn the phone off. Focus your mind on the exercises; block out all distractions, mentally and physically.

EYE EXERCISE PROTOCOL

Practice these eye exercise techniques two or three times a week. The day after your first eye routine your eye muscles may be sore; do not worry, this soreness will gradually leave. Soreness means that you have "worked-out" weak eye muscles that have been lying dormant, perhaps for many years. They are resilient and, like your arm muscles, will respond with renewed vigor.

Take a one, two, or three day rest between each eye session, depending on your energy level. The rest period between each eye exercise session is as important as the eye exercises. During periods of rest the eyes and body heal and rebuild, imparting strength and health. Performing eye exercises too often can easily cause eyestrain, which is a basic reason why most eye routines fail. The eye exercises that follow, if practiced regularly and consistently, can help bring your vision back to 20–20 and beyond. Perform the eye exercises with joy and relaxation. Results will be forthcoming.

Important Eye Training Note: Always remove your glasses when performing vision exercises—it gives the eyes full flexibility. If you are able to move around without your glasses, do so when you start this program; otherwise wear them during your daily activities. As your eyesight improves visit your eye doctor to be fitted for weaker eyeglass lenses. Be persistent and your vision will improve.

 Lazy Eight Neck Loosening Exercise
(Pre–Eye Exercise Warm-Up Technique)

The Lazy Eight exercise is performed first in your routine because it relaxes your neck muscles and allows fresh blood to flow to the eyes and brain. It prepares you for the rest of your eye routine and ensures greater success in improving your vision.

1. To perform the Lazy Eight exercise, simply draw imaginary

"figure eights" with your nose, moving your head slowly and smoothly. This will loosen the back of your neck, calm your nervous system, and enable you to focus your eyes clearly. Large "figure eights" help to relax the larger muscles of the eyes, while tiny "figure eights" relax the smaller muscles of the eyes.

2. Vary the "figure eights" by drawing them vertically, then horizontally. Perform them right to left and left to right, then top to bottom and bottom to top. Spend at least three minutes on this exercise.

 ## Eye Exercise 1:
Egyptian Black Dot Technique

(Eye Muscle Exercise)

The Egyptian Black Dot technique is one of the most important exercises for all eye conditions.

First prepare your black dot on a 2" x 3" white card. Draw a black dot about the size of a dime on the card with black ink. If you have trouble seeing up close (farsightedness), do not perform the first part of the Black Dot technique. Perform the second part only.

⊚ Egyptian Black Dot Technique—Part I: Straight in Front

1. Hold the card in front of your eyes at arm's length (see fig. 4.1 on page 50).
2. Next, move card to the tip of your nose. Do not move your head; move the card only. Gaze at the black dot for 30 seconds. You must see only one dot; this means that both eyes are working together. If you see two dots, move the card away from your nose until you see one dot.
3. After 30 seconds move the card straight out in front of your eyes, then rest and close your eyes for a few seconds.

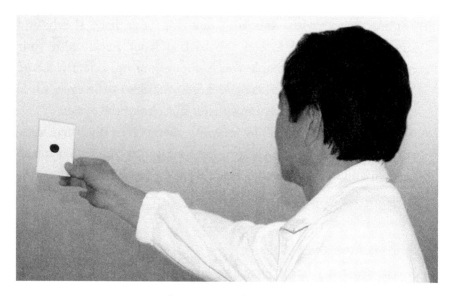

Fig. 4.1. The Egyptian Black Dot Technique

4. Next, raise the card up between your eyebrows and gaze at the dot for 30 seconds. Move the card as close as you can while seeing only one dot. Rest for a few seconds.

Be persistent and consistent and you will see results. Remember to breathe gently, deeply, and naturally.

❂ Egyptian Black Dot Technique—Part II: To the Right and Left

1. While keeping your head straight, move the black dot to your right shoulder and gaze at it for 30 seconds.
2. Then, move the dot to your left shoulder and gaze at it for 30 seconds. Close eyes and rest.

Farsighted people can perform this shoulder-to-shoulder Black Dot exercise with great benefit. The Egyptian Black Dot techniques make the eye muscles focus in positions in which they do not normally focus. This helps to reshape and balance the eyeball itself.

Eye Exercise 2:
Egyptian Letter Gazing Technique

(Eye Muscle Exercise for Close and Distant Vision)

Preschool children naturally look in all directions with their eyes. Then school children are taught to look directly ahead and down at their books. After many years of these poor eye habits, they stop looking in all directions, and the eyeball loses its natural shape. Consequently, vision problems result.

The Egyptian Letter Gazing Technique enables the eyes to focus in all directions and allows both eyes to see together. It also helps to reshape the eye in its normal position, so that light can focus on the retina properly for perfect eyesight. This technique coordinates the mind and eyes so that they work in perfect harmony. Practice will bring improvement. Stick with it! Persistence is the key to success in vision improvement.

Basic Egyptian Letter Gazing Technique

Cut out three ⅛" to ¼" thick letters from a newspaper or magazine and glue them on a 2" × 3" white card.

Perform each movement with one eye at a time, then use both eyes together. The eye that is covered with your palm is to be kept open during the exercise. This enables both eyes to work together during the exercise. Start out with 3 repetitions in each direction (see fig. 4.2 on page 52). Every 2 to 3 weeks add 1 repetition, until you reach 6 repetitions.

1. **First Movement:** Hold the card 12 inches in front of your eyes. Concentrate on one of the letters, always focusing to see it clearly. Move the card above the eyes and below the chin 3 times. Do this one eye at a time and then both eyes together. Keep your head still—move your eyes only.
2. **Second Movement:** Hold the card 12 inches in front of your eyes.

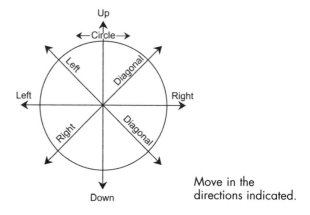

Move in the directions indicated.

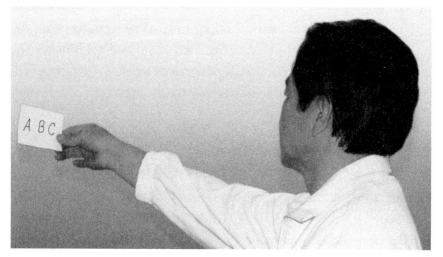

Fig. 4.2. The Egyptian Letter Gazing Technique

Concentrate on one of the letters, always focusing to see it clearly. Move the card slowly from your right eye to your left eye—always keeping sight of the letters. Perform with one eye, then both eyes together, 3 times each.

3. **Third Movement:** Hold the letters in front of your face. Concentrate on one of the letters, always focusing to see it clearly, while moving the card to the right and left diagonally. Perform 3 times each way. Again, work with one eye at a time, then both together.

4. **Fourth Movement:** Concentrate on one of the letters, always focusing to see it clearly, while moving the card in large circles, at arm's length. Perform 3 times each way, one eye at a time, then both together.

5. **Fifth Movement:** Concentrate on one of the letters, always focusing to see it clearly, while holding the card about 12 inches in front of your head and then moving it smoothly in a 10-inch diameter circle. Perform 10 times clockwise and 10 times counterclockwise. Perform with one eye at a time, and both eyes together.

Important Note: Breathe deeply and naturally and try not to blink. See the letter as clearly as possible without eyestrain. These Egyptian eye techniques are superior exercises for reshaping the eyeballs and strengthening the eye muscles. They help to create eye muscle balance. Do not confuse these exercises with ordinary eye exercises—there is no comparison!

Advanced Egyptian Letter Gazing Technique

After practicing the Basic Egyptian Letter Gazing technique with a card 1 foot in front of your eyes for a month, you will be ready to practice the Advanced Egyptian Letter Gazing technique.

Paste a black letter on a 2" × 3" card and tape the card to one end of a 12-inch ruler, with the card perpendicular to the ruler and the letter facing you. The letter should be big enough for you to see easily at 2 feet. Hold the card at least 2 to 3 feet from your eyes. To overcome myopia (nearsightedness), you must use your eyes to see beyond 2 feet. As your eyesight becomes clear at this distance, you can use smaller letters to help you obtain further improvement.

To improve your close vision (farsightedness), simply perform the eye exercise while holding the letters less than 12 inches from your eyes. Perform this advanced exercise in the same sequence as you did in the above basic technique.

Important Note for Egyptian Black Letter Technique: Be sure you can see the letter sharp and clear! Use a black letter that you can see clearly. Take your time in moving the card closer or further. For example, bring the card "in" 1 inch only every few weeks for close vision (farsightedness). The same holds true for distant vision (nearsightedness)—move it only an inch or two at a time every few weeks. Don't be in a hurry to force your eyes to see better.

 Eye Exercise 3:
Yoga Accommodative Eye Exercises
(To Improve Close and Distant Vision)

Modern science tells us that the accommodative eye muscles weaken with age. However, this is not universally true. The accommodative eye muscles, just like any other body muscles, become weaker, not as a result of age, but of disuse. If you continue to use the accommodative focusing eye muscles regularly, your eyesight will remain clear and strong throughout life. Think of this: when you regularly perform arm, chest, and back exercises with weights or machines, your muscles grow strong. What works for one kind of muscle, physiologically, bio-logically, and mechanically, will work for all. Eye exercises foster fresh blood flow, chi flow, and nerve force to the eye muscles and nerves, thereby enhancing vision.

The ancient Hindu yogis devised many techniques for improving eyesight. This marvelous eye exercise helps the eyes to improve their ability to change focus and see clearly in the distance and at the close point. It also prevents the accommodative muscles from weakening. If you have lost this accommodative eye focusing ability, this eye exer-cise can bring back your natural eye accommodation and regain the muscles' elasticity. Perform it 2 or 3 times a week.

Practice the Yoga Accommodative Eye Exercise xercise outside in good light or inside in a well-lighted room, while looking out the window.

✪ Yoga Accommodative Eye Exercise—Part I

1. Pick out a distant object, about 20 feet or more away (such as a tree, car, or building). This is your distant vision object.
2. In your hand, hold a 2" × 3" card with black letters, large enough for you to see clearly.
3. Hold the card at eye level at arm's length away, or where you can see a given letter on the card clearly (fig. 4.3). This is your close point object.
4. Look at a distant object; see it clearly. Now, move your eyes back to a letter on the card and see it clearly for a few seconds. Perform this accommodative eye movement 3 times (in and out).
5. When the letter on the card becomes easier to see, then move the card a couple inches closer; then repeat the movement between the distant point and close point 3 times, as in step 4.
6. Next, move the card a few inches closer, while still seeing it clearly. Again, repeat the distant and close eye movement, always focusing your eyes as clearly as you can.

Practice this exercise one eye at a time, then with both eyes together. Eventually, you'll be able to see the letters on the card at the close point, 4 or 5 inches from your eyes, clear and sharp.

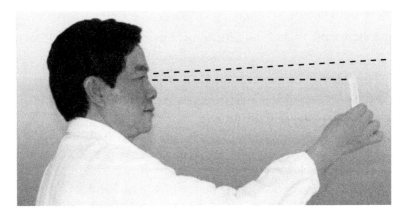

Fig. 4.3. A black letter on the card serves as your close point object
for the Yoga Accomodative Eye Exercise.

Yoga Accommodative Eye Exercise—Part II
(To Improve Distant Vision)

Follow the steps in Part I, but reverse the procedure by looking at a card with letters on it, held at reading distance, 15 to 18 inches away from your eyes.

1. Hold the card where you are able to see the letters clearly, then immediately look at any object 20 feet away, such as a tree, car, or building.
2. Next, focus your eyes from the card to the distant object, seeing both as clearly as possible; look back and forth 3 times.
3. Next, look at an object 20 to 30 feet farther away than the first object. Repeat the back and forth eye movement 3 times.

Continue with this exercise as you look at objects farther into the distance. Practice this distance-seeing accommodative eye movement for 5 minutes, 2 or 3 times a week.

Eye Exercise 4: Tai Chi Rocker Eye Technique
(To Improve Close and Distant Vision)

While studying and practicing Chi Kung and Tai Chi exercises, I (Mantak Chia) made an amazing discovery of a new way to improve the eyesight with a Chi Kung movement called the Tai Chi Rocker. It is an invaluable eye exercise to improve both close and distant vision. Just a few minutes of the Tai Chi Rocker eye technique will give your eyes a thorough workout and strengthen your eye focusing muscles. Tai Chi Rocker also relaxes the eyes, as well as centering and grounding the mind, body, and spirit. Practice this exercise for 5 to 10 minutes, 2 or 3 times a week.

1. Place Chart 1, the Snellen Eye Chart, on the wall at eye level (see Chart 1 on page 57). Shine a bright light on the chart to prevent eyestrain.

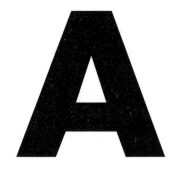

A

C G Fifty Feet

Thirty Feet

F E P Twenty Feet

L Z O D Fifteen Feet

C N G A B Ten Feet

H A Q O E Five Feet

Z U K L T P A Three Feet

B R O C G D N Two Feet

Chart 1. The Snellen Eye Chart

2. Stand 2 or 3 feet away from the chart. Place your right foot 6 inches in front of the left. Gaze at one of the letters on the chart that you can see easily.

3. To start, begin to rock back and forth. When rocking backward the front right foot lifts up and the back foot stays flat on the ground. While rocking forward the back of the left foot lifts up, while the front right foot stays on the ground (fig. 4.4). Rock back and forth for 1 or 2 minutes. Relax, and allow the letter on the chart to become clear in your vision.

4. Next, switch the position of your feet. Place your left foot forward and the right foot behind you. Practice the rocking movement for 1 to 2 minutes.

This exercise can be used to improve both distance vision and

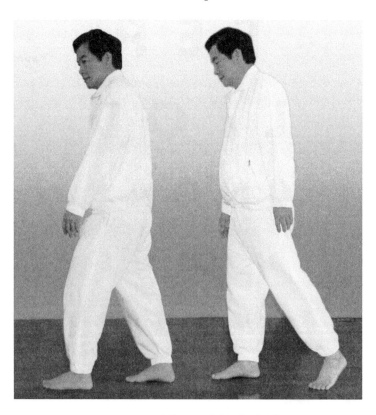

Fig. 4.4. As you rock forward, lift the left heel up.

close vision. For close vision improvement only, rock within 2 feet of the chart; do not move further back. To improve your distant vision, you can move back as far as you can see the letters on the chart—5 to 60 feet away.

Every 2 to 3 minutes, close your eyes and relax your body. Feel your eyes becoming softer and more relaxed. Also, remember the black letter clearly in your mind. For best results, close your eyes and place both palms over the eyes for 15 seconds (see Palming technique, chapter 2).

Vital Points to Remember While Performing the Tai Chi Rocker Eye Technique

Point 1: To improve close vision, rock toward the chart and stop rocking forward as soon as the letter on the chart starts to blur, then rock back.

Point 2: To improve distant vision, move further away from the chart. Imagine pulling the letters out of the eye chart as you rock backward. As you rock forward, notice the letter becoming clearer.

Point 3: Remember to perform the Palming technique every two minutes; try to soften and relax your eyes and mind.

Point 4: Shine a bright light on the eye chart to prevent eyestrain. Or perform the eye exercises in natural outdoor light.

Point 5: Focus on the eye chart letters with a soft, relaxed gaze.

Point 6: Never hold your breath—breathe deeply and gently.

Point 7: Practice with one eye at a time. Place your palm over one eye while both eyes are open—this enables both eyes to work together. Finally, practice with both eyes together.

After performing the Tai Chi Rocker, perform yoga stretching movements. Reach for the sky with both hands and one hand at a time, bend over and touch your toes; stretch backward, to the sides; roll your neck in circles. Stretching releases tension, and improves blood and nerve circulation to the eyes. (See the Internal Chi Kung energy exercises in chapter 5.)

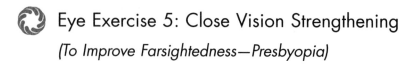

Eye Exercise 5: Close Vision Strengthening
(To Improve Farsightedness—Presbyopia)

Close Vision Technique A: Whipping

Whipping is an exercise that greatly helps presbyopia (middle-age sight), farsightedness, and any other close vision problems. It is one of the best eye exercises for strengthening the accommodative eye muscles to improve close vision.

1. Cup your left palm over your left eye.
2. Hold a card with a black letter on it that you can easily see at arm's length in front of your eyes.
3. Pull the card toward your right eye at a moderate speed until it is within a few inches of your face.
4. Next, quickly "whip" the card suddenly back to arm's length. Repeat this movement several times.
5. Then, do the same thing using the left eye while the right eye is cupped with your right palm. Repeat several times.
6. Next, practice Whipping with both eyes open at the same time. Repeat several times.

Perform this exercise 2 to 3 times a week.

Close Vision Technique B: Tromboning

1. Hold a card with a small black letter on it that you can easily see at arm's length.
2. From arm's length, "slide" (move) the card 3 inches toward your right eye, then move it back to arm's length.
3. Next, slide the card 6 inches toward your right eye, then move it back out to arm's length.

4. Next, slide the card 9 inches toward your right eye, then move it back out to arm's length.

5. Progress in this manner 3 inches at a time until the card is a couple inches away from your eye. Practice this sequence several times with your right eye.

6. Next, perform Tromboning with your left eye, then with both eyes together.

Move the card at a moderate easy speed. Relax and breathe easily. After practicing this exercise for a few weeks, vary the speed of the card—sometimes moving the card more slowly, other times at a brisk speed. Consistently practiced, Whipping and Tromboning eventually awaken and strengthen the focusing muscles for the close point, until you will be able to see the print sharply and clearly.

◎ Close Vision Technique C: Close Point Eye Sharpening Technique

Many people go through middle age with blurry vision at the close point. This does not have to happen. You can do something about it. This exercise, together with the previous one, will help you to strengthen and improve your close vision.

I (Mantak Chia) have found that, performed correctly, this Close Point Eye Sharpening technique is the most important eye technique to improve close vision. It is easy to do and only needs to be practiced twice a week. I devised this eye improvement technique in 1995. It is done by tracing letters on the chart. Tracing is looking at the whole letter, or going over the letter like you are tracing or coloring it on a paper. This is different from tracking or edging, which is going around the edge of the letter or other object.

(See Chart 2. Close Vision, Principles of Eye Training, on page 63.)

1. Hold Chart 2 in front of your eyes, from 12 to 20 inches away, where you can see it without strain.
2. Trace the first letter of the first paragraph with your eyes, that is, the *V* in "Vision."
3. Close your eyes and trace and visualize the letter in your mind.
4. Open your eyes, look at the letter, and trace it again.
5. Close your eyes and trace the letter again, then open your eyes while inhaling and exhaling a gentle deep breath, and look at the letter.
6. Slowly move the chart in toward your eyes while trying to see the letter as clearly as possible—when the letter starts to blur, stop the movement (fig. 4.5).
7. Close your eyes for a few seconds. Open your eyes with a deep breath and move the chart away from your eyes, and notice the letter become clearer.
8. Place both palms over the eyes for 20 seconds, while visualizing a black color.

Repeat steps 1 through 8 with the first letter of all eleven paragraphs, for example, the letter *T* for paragraph 2, *R* for paragraph 3, and so forth. Or go down to the smallest paragraph that you can see clearly. Practice this exercise at least 15 to 20 minutes, 2 or 3 times a week.

Move the letter away from your eyes and notice it becoming clearer.

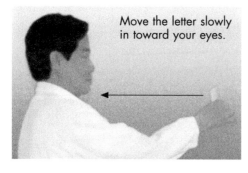
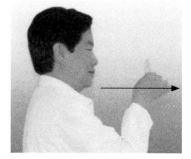

Fig. 4.5. Close Vision Technique C—Close Point Eye Sharpening Technique

CHART 2. CLOSE VISION
Principles of Eye Training

1. Vision can be improved by natural methods.

2. Tension causes eyestrain and impairs vision. Relaxation relieves tension.

3. Relaxed eyes are normal eyes. When eyes lose their relaxation and become tense, they strain and stare and the vision becomes poor.

4. Vision can be improved only by education in proper seeing. Proper seeing is relaxed seeing. Normal eyes shift rapidly and continuously. Eyes with defective vision become fixed and staring. When staring eyes learn to shift, vision improves.

5. The eyeball is like the camera, and changes in focal length. To focus the camera, you must adjust the distance from the film to the front of the camera.

6. To focus the eye, the distance between the retina at the back and the cornea in front must be increased for close vision and decreased for distant vision.

7. Six muscles on the outside of the eyeball control its shape; four, reaching from front to back, flatten the eye; two, belting it around the middle, squeeze and lengthen it from front to back.

8. When the eyes are relaxed, these six muscles are flexible and cooperate automatically, adjusting the focal length so eyes may see both near and far.

9. Just as dependence on crutches weakens leg muscles, so dependence on glasses weakens eye muscles by relieving them of responsibility. But muscles can be reeducated to do their duties.

10. Relaxation of the eyes and mind brings relaxation of the entire body. This general relaxation increases circulation and brings improved physical, visual, and mental health.

11. Relaxation is a sensation.

Eye Exercise 6: Stretch Your Vision

(Distance Vision Strengthening Exercise to Improve Nearsightedness)

This exercise was taught in Michigan, in the 1940s, by two optometrists, Drs. Ross and Rhymer. It is extremely valuable in extending the limits of your distance vision, especially for myopic vision (nearsightedness).

To start, place the Snellen Eye Chart (page 57) on a wall at eye level, with a good light shining on it.

1. Stand straight and select one of the letters on the chart.
2. Trace your chosen letter in your mind, then close your eyes for a few seconds. Relax your hands, shoulders, eyes, legs, neck, and so forth (fig. 4.6).
3. Open your eyes and look at the letter again.
4. Next, place both palms over your eyes and Palm while visualizing the letter in your mind for 15 seconds (fig. 4.7).
5. Open your eyes with a deep inhalation and exhalation of breath, noticing the letter becoming blacker.
6. While looking at the letter, begin swaying slowly from side to

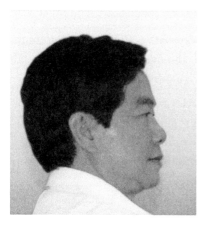

1) Look at chart and trace one letter.
2) Close eyes, relax body.
3) Open eyes and look at letter.

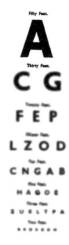

Fig. 4.6. Stretch Your Vision

side. While you continue to sway, move s-l-o-w-l-y away from the chart, taking very short backward steps. Breathe naturally and allow the print to come in clearly. When you reach the point where the print becomes indistinct or unreadable, STOP! At this point, bend forward at the waist, continuing to sway, and again read the letter. Now, resume your short backward steps.

Even though you are leaning far forward, you will again reach a point at which the printed letters will no longer be legible. When this occurs, straighten up, move close to the chart and repeat the exercise on the next smaller line, following the above instructions. Repeat each line until you reach the bottom line of the chart.

It is important to relax the entire body while performing this exercise. Mentally and physically feel your shoulders, neck, face, eye, arms, and hands relax. Let go of your jaw muscles and let them drop. Let your eyes become soft and calm. Practice Stretch Your Vision at least 15 to 30 minutes, 2 or 3 times a week.

Important Note on Lighting: When performing this exercise inside, be sure a bright light shines on your Snellen Eye Chart to prevent eyestrain. Use a 150- to 200-watt bulb or a bright floodlight.

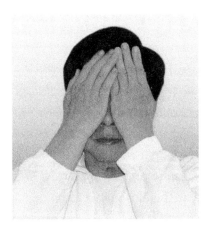

1) Palm 20 seconds.
2) Open eyes with deep breath.
3) Look at letter and walk backward.

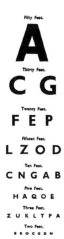

Fig. 4.7. Palming while visualizing the letter

Eye Exercise 7: Test Card Eye Exercise

(To Improve Close and Distant Vision)

Dr. Bates recommended this eye exercise to help strengthen distant and close vision. It can be performed during your regular routine, or during spare moments throughout the day. It is also a great eye exercise for those who have already achieved good eyesight, and want to maintain their excellent vision.

Close Vision Exercise

Stand 2 feet away from the Snellen Eye Chart (see page 57).

1. Look at the top letter—*A*—on the eye chart and trace it with your eyes or nose.
2. Close your eyes for 5 seconds. Relax eyes and open them with a gentle breath, and notice the letter *A* appearing blacker and clearer.
3. Palm your eyes for 20 seconds. Open eyes with a gentle breath, and notice the letter appearing blacker and clearer.
4. Look at the next line on the eye chart, with the letters *C* and *G*. Repeat the above sequence.

Perform these four steps all the way down to the bottom line on the chart. When you can clearly see the bottom line, move 3 inches closer to the chart. Each week move closer, but do not be in any hurry to do this if you cannot see the letters clearly. In other words, move closer *only* when the letters come in clearly. Never strain to see the letters on the eye chart. However, when you are working with the larger letters on the upper lines you can move closer to the chart even if you cannot see the smaller letters on the lower lines. Move closer to the upper larger lines that you can see clearly.

The goal is to read the smallest line at 4 or 5 inches away. If you can do this, you'll have perfect eyesight at the close point. Practice 2 or 3 times weekly, until you achieve this goal. If one eye is stronger than the other, put an eye patch on the stronger eye and go through this routine looking only with the weak eye. Just play with it and you will be delighted with the results.

Distance Vision Exercise

Stand 6 to 12 inches away from the Snellen Eye Chart (page 57).

1. Look at the top letter—*A*—on the eye chart and trace and track it with your eyes or nose.
2. Close your eyes for 5 seconds. Relax eyes and open them with a gentle breath, and notice the letter *A* appearing blacker and clearer.
3. Palm your eyes for 20 seconds. Open eyes with a gentle breath, and notice the letter appearing blacker and clearer.
4. Look at the next line on the eye chart, with the letters *C* and *G*. Repeat the above sequence.

Perform these four steps all the way down to the bottom line on the Snellen Eye Chart. When you can see the bottom line, move 1 foot further away from the chart. Each week move farther back, but do not be in any hurry to do this if you cannot see the letters clearly. In other words, move further back *only* when the letters come in clearly. Never strain to see the letters on the eye chart. However, you can move further back when working with the top five lines on the chart, even if you cannot see the smaller letters on the lower lines. Move further back while working with the upper larger letters you can see clearly.

Eye Exercise 8:
Tibetan Peripheral Vision Technique

How important is peripheral vision? Everyone uses their peripheral vision while driving, walking, playing sports, at work, and at home. In fact, if we didn't use our peripheral vision, we would develop "tunnel vision," just like the old gray mare going down the street with blinders attached to the sides of her eyes. She can only look forward and is blind to everything else around her.

Before being taught to read, children have sharp peripheral vision. We gradually lose our capacity for clear peripheral vision by concentrating with a fixed hard gaze straight in front of us. But we can regain that ability. Great sports athletes like Wayne Gretsky, Barry Sanders, and Michael Jordan are praised by their peers for having "eyes at the back of their heads." They know where the ball or puck is at every moment. They have developed extremely good peripheral vision.

By developing your peripheral vision, you too can have "eyes at the back of your head." With strong, well-developed side vision, you can prevent accidents while driving. Your ability to play any sport will improve dramatically.

1. Hold a pencil in each hand, 12 inches in front of your eyes (fig. 4.8). Look straight forward, without moving your head or your gaze to

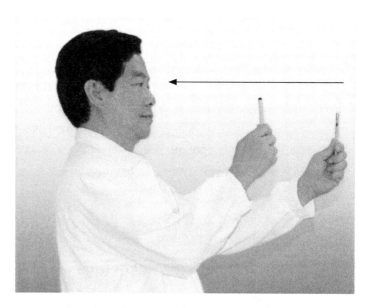

Fig. 4.8. Tibetan Peripheral Vision Technique

either side. Keep your eyes looking straight ahead throughout the exercise.

2. Gaze straight out past the pencils into the distance, without looking directly at the pencils, while continuing to be aware of them.

3. Move each pencil s-l-o-w-l-y to the side of your head, as far as you can see it peripherally. Repeat this front-to-side movement at least 10 times on each side.

4. Next, move the pencils, right hand upward and left hand downward, 10 times.

5. Then reverse this motion with the left hand moving upward and right hand moving downward, 10 times.

6. Next, while holding the pencils 12 inches away, move your right hand diagonally upward and left hand diagonally downward 10 times.

7. Next, move your left hand diagonally upward and right hand diagonally downward 10 times.

8. Next, with the pencils 12 inches in front of your eyes, simultaneously move each pencil in a circle about 2 or 3 feet in diameter from the center out to the side. Perform circles clockwise and counterclockwise.

Important Eye Training Note: Allow your side vision to come into focus naturally without effort. Do not strain to see peripherally. When you walk, drive, or read, use your peripheral vision to see the buildings, cars, furniture, and people around you. Blocking out the side vision creates eye muscle imbalance and is a major cause of imperfect eyesight. Many accidents can be prevented with well-developed peripheral vision. Practice the Tibetan Peripheral Vision technique 3 to 5 minutes, 2 to 3 times a week.

Eye Exercise 9:
Yoga Eye-Palming Techniques

(Always finish eye exercises with Palming)

Prior to the rediscovery of Palming by Dr. Bates in the early 1900s, eye-palming techniques were practiced by ancient Indian yogis and Chinese Taoists for thousands of years. They practiced Palming as a form of meditation or inner visualization and relaxation. According to the masters, too much outward gazing at all the exciting, bright, and fast-moving things in the world upsets the inner balance of our spiritual third eye. Our physical eyes and brain become clouded, confused, and agitated, like a muddy stream. Palming calms our mind, emotions, spirit, and body. Our inner and outer eyes take on the qualities of a clear, tranquil, peaceful pool of water. When our mind is tranquil, our eyesight focuses on the world with clarity and insight.

The yogis of India discovered that performing Palming in the fetal kneeling position or fetal squatting position is more healing than in the upright sitting position. However, all three Palming positions are beneficial and can be performed at any time.

The Yoga Fetal Palming Technique

Performing Palming in the fetal kneeling or squatting position is an excellent method of complete eye, mind, and body relaxation. Fresh blood circulation and nerve flow to the eyes are also greatly enhanced.

Kneeling Fetal Position Palming Technique

While kneeling in the fetal position (on knees, with body bent forward, face down), bring your head to the floor in front of your knees, with your palms cupped over your eyes. Rest the heels of your palms on your cheekbones, and cross your fingers over your forehead. Be sure your palms do not touch your eyeballs; keep out as much light as possible. Visualize black velvet.

○ Squatting Fetal Position Palming Technique

Squat down with feet 8 to 10 inches apart. Place your arms over your knees and cup your palms over your eyes. Relax in this position with palms covering eyes. In the East people squat in this position to have babies, eat, and eliminate. It is a natural position and very conducive to relaxation, meditation, and Palming.

◉ *Seated Palming Technique*

Place your palms over your eyes, elbows on table, with back and neck straight. You can use a small pillow under your elbows if you wish; this helps to relax your arms. Use this method at work if you are unable to perform the Fetal Palming technique. (You wouldn't want to be caught on the floor when your boss walks in!)

◉ *Let Go Mentally While Palming*

While Palming, let go mentally. Your eyes cannot completely relax when the mind or body is full of stress and tension. The brain is like a camera—we see through the brain. If your brain is tense, thinking about your problems, you can strain your eyes while Palming, just as you can strain them while they are open. You must relax your "brain-stuff" (thoughts) while Palming. Then you will experience improved eyesight.

For complete relaxation, breathe slowly, evenly, and naturally. Give your problems to the universe or Higher Power. Let your mind dwell on something beautiful such as a blue ocean, sandy beach, sunset, mountains, or a loving face. Complete relaxation leads to complete healing—this is your goal!

◉ *Key to Seeing Perfect Blackness*

To see the fullest degree of blackness, first look at a perfectly black object, such as a black car, black cat or dog, or black velvet. Then (while Palming) try to remember that blackness. Perfect blackness that is recalled and perceived indicates that the mind is perfectly relaxed. When you cultivate the power to "remember black," your brain and mind will be relaxed and rested instantaneously, and your eyesight strengthened tremendously.

Your mastery in remembering to see black goes beyond relaxation. It enables you to see the letters on a page much blacker, thus making them sharper and easier to read. Practice a few minutes each day and you will see marked improvement. Your subconscious memory of perfect blackness, carried in your mind when your eyes are open, will give you a high degree of mental and visual clarity and strength. Thus, your vision can be improved immediately.

◎ Secret Black Globe Palming Technique

The real inner secret behind perfect eyesight is to relax the eyes, body, brain, and mind completely! To do this, you must be able to visualize totally black space while Palming with your eyes closed. When you think that you have pictured a background as black as it can be, imagine a very black globe pictured against that background. What do you see? You will see something still blacker than the background. Then let go of the background and let the black globe spread out until it becomes the background itself.

Try to picture a still blacker globe on the new background and so on, until you get a background so black that nothing blacker can be imagined. Perfect blackness equals perfect relaxation, and perfect relaxation equals perfect vision.

Ten to 15 minutes of seeing black while Palming will prove to you what a marvelous relaxation technique this is. Some people have reported that their eyestrain was relieved in only a few Palming sessions. After seeing black, you will be able to see much more clearly and strongly—at both the close point and far point.

Important Eye Improvement Note: When you Palm correctly, you will see perfect blackness. The blacker you see while Palming, the faster your eyesight will improve. Perfect blackness indicates that your visual nerves are relaxed and functioning correctly. If you see gray or various colors while Palming, it indicates that your vision is unclear and blurry. However, don't try to force blackness in the "Palming field area." That will only cause more tension and weak vision. When your inner mind is able to see, visualize, and remember *black* while Palming, your vision will improve.

For best results in eye improvement, practice Palming every single day. If you make time for your Palming exercise, time will be good to your eyes in your golden years. Bates and other natural eye training specialists state that many cases of imperfect eyesight—nearsightedness, farsightedness, aging vision—have been permanently cured by the simple practice of seeing black while Palming over a period of time.

After each eye exercise session, Palm for at least 5 minutes. Relax! After Palming, open your eyes and notice how the trees, grass, sky, houses, and people appear clear, bright, and more colorful. Happy Palming!

❷ *Heal Liver and Eyes with the Color of Green*

In the Orient, the Taoist masters teach that the color green is associated with the liver and the eyes. Green vegetables and nature's green colors, such as trees and grass, help to heal the liver and also heal your eyes too! So, while Palming, you can sometimes visualize green trees, green grass, or blue-green ocean to help your eyes and mind become calmer, happier, and more peaceful.

PROGRESSIVE EYE TRAINING

Chapter 9 provides some suggested eye exercise routines, but in general, follow these recommendations for progressive eye training: each month make your eye routine more progressive and challenging; perform more repetitions; stand farther away from the eye chart; increase

Palming time and frequency; change your eye routine or perform different eye exercises for your specific eye condition.

Progressive eye training exercises increase circulation to the eyes for quicker eye improvement. If your eyes get overly sore or fatigued from eye training, take a break from your eye routine for a couple days to allow nerve, tendon, and eye muscle healing and repair.

Always move your eyes smoothly during your eye muscle exercises. Smooth eye movements relax the eyes, which helps you to see clearly. Keep practicing until you perform all eye routines smoothly and calmly. When you reach perfect eyesight—20–10 or better—a fifteen-minute eye routine, once a week, is enough to maintain perfect vision. Also, continue your daily natural eye habits for life. You can prevent eye problems and maintain perfect eyesight for as long as you live. Be healthy and prosper!

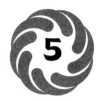

Vision Improvement through Healing the Kidneys and Liver

ORIENTAL EYE AND HEALTH DIAGNOSIS

The eyes are the mirror of physical health. The human eye holds many inner secrets. Oriental herbal doctors report that the eyes operate in close connection with the liver. A poorly functioning liver causes the eyes to ache and creates dark circles around them that do not bear the light very well.

Jean Rofidel, a master of Do-In (self-massage) says: "The eyes of a person in good health bear everything—blinding light, cold and wind, onions, and so on—without crying." Thus, if you are in good health you do not need sunglasses. Rofidel continues: "If you blink too much (more than three times a minute), it is a sign of organic weakness [especially of the liver]."

The consumption of too many sweets, fats, animal foods, and alcohol makes the eyes tired and weak. Sexual excess causes dark circles around the eyes. Excess liquid intake causes waterlogged kidneys, edema, weakness, lower back pain, excess eye blinking, and puffy bags under the eyes.

Traditional Chinese doctors say that the kidneys are the mother organs of the body. They regulate water and protein. Too much or not enough of each can result in poor health and illness. Strong kidneys impart calmness to the mind and spirit. Weak kidneys instill fear and trembling throughout the body, mind, and spirit. Healthy kidneys nourish the liver, so they contribute indirectly to improved eyesight.

INTERNAL CHI KUNG ENERGY EXERCISES FOR VISION IMPROVEMENT

Good posture and internal organ health is vitally important for clear sharp vision. The yogis and Chi Kung masters practice stretching and posture exercises to strengthen their kidneys and lower back area. The kidneys are considered the health and longevity organs of the body. If you want to stay young, vibrant, and full of energy, practice these internal exercises daily.

These powerful exercise movements have been taught and practiced throughout the world in every culture.

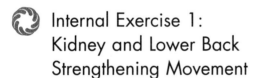 Internal Exercise 1: Kidney and Lower Back Strengthening Movement

This exercise will help to strengthen your kidneys and lower back.

1. Stand with feet close together.
2. Reach forward, without bending the knees; look upward with your eyes and bend forward while trying to touch the floor with your hands (fig. 5.1). Feel the stretch in your lower back. Looking up keeps your back straight. This movement normalizes the lower back, strengthens the kidneys, and helps you to stay grounded and balanced. Perform 6 times.

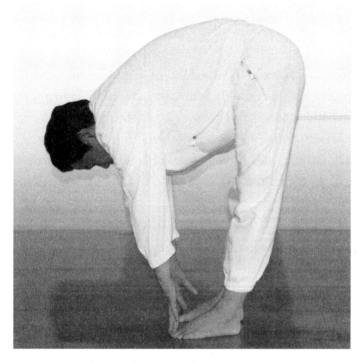

Fig. 5.1. Kidney and Lower Back Strengthening Movement

 Internal Exercise 2:
Spine Straightening Movement

Good posture is the key to good energy circulation to the eyes and the organs that nourish the eyes. This simple exercise is invaluable for improving and maintaining a healthy, strong posture for life.

Simply let your head fall backward while standing in an upright posture. Hold this position for 15 seconds. Perform this movement several times a day. It straightens the spine and raises the chest. Your body becomes gracefully poised, with a straight posture. This posture enables your lungs to expand and breathe more deeply; it makes it easier for the blood to circulate through the heart and imparts more confidence.

Internal Exercise 3:
Reaching for Heaven

This movement benefits the eyesight, ears, and complexion; increases lung capacity and respiration; stimulates the liver, kidneys, stomach, intestines, and colon; helps to overcome constipation; improves sex gland function; trims, tones, strengthens, and flattens the abdomen; overcomes fatigue; and increases energy. Stretch up to the sky and watch your energy zoom!

1. Stand with your feet 12 inches apart, with arms in front of your body and fingers intertwined.
2. Inhale a gentle deep breath while lifting your arms up above your head, turning your palms to face up, and stretching up on your toes (fig. 5.2). You can keep your head forward or, for variation, look upward at your hands.

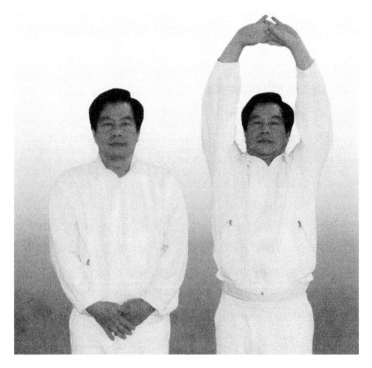

Fig. 5.2. Reaching for Heaven

3. Then, hold your breath and stretch your arms upward and hold for a few seconds.

4. Exhale; lower your arms down sideways. This movement helps to remove the "hump" out of the upper back and straightens the spine and posture. This natural upward stretch breaks up blockages in the body for improved circulation and greater health. Repeat 6 times.

 ## Internal Exercise 4: Tibetan Rejuvenation Rite

The Tibetan Rejuvenation Rite comes from the Tibetan monks high up in the Himalayan mountains in northern India. This powerful "rite" strengthens the back and shoulder muscles. It also strengthens the neck and leg areas; increases blood and nerve circulation to the brain and vital internal organs; helps to overcome constipation; slows down the aging process; increases lung capacity and breathing ability; trims, tones, and firms the waist and buttocks; helps improve blood and nerve circulation to the eyes.

1. Lie on your stomach and place hands on the floor, shoulder-width apart.

2. Next, push upper body (shoulders and head) up and back, with hips almost touching the floor. Stretch neck and upper body as far back as possible (see fig. 5.3 on p. 80).

3. From this position, raise up on your toes and hands, while lifting your hips straight up, pointing the top of your head to the floor, and touching your chin to your chest.

Breathe in as your hips are raised, and breathe out when raising your head. Start with 6 repetitions and work up to 15 or 20. You'll feel invigorated and full of chi!

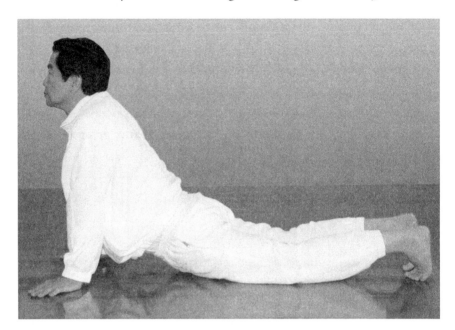

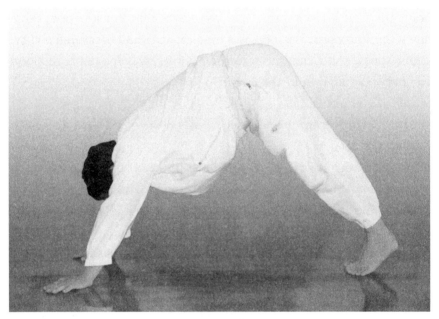

Fig. 5.3. The Tibetan Rejuvenation Rite

Internal Exercise 5:
Sufi Bear Walk (Egyptian)

Perform this "walk" for a minute at least 3 times per week. After doing it for a month, add 1 minute each month until you are walking on all fours for 3 minutes. The Sufi Bear Walk strengthens the nerves and allows fresh blood to circulate directly to the eyes and brain. It tones the shoulder, back, arm, and leg muscles. When you "walk" fast, you'll increase your endurance and stamina. Bears have a straight and powerful posture. This exercise rebuilds postural muscles and overcomes the downward gravitational pull, which helps to overcome falling organs. It also imparts an internal massage to the abdomen and colon, thus helping to alleviate constipation and gastrointestinal problems.

This exercise takes some practice to perform correctly. It is done by using all four limbs in a "cross-crawl" fashion like a bear, dog, or cat. While "walking" on all fours (hands and feet), move your right arm and left leg forward at the same time, then your left arm and right leg. Using opposite arms and legs activates the right and left hemispheres of the brain, bringing balance and harmony to the body/mind connection.

 Internal Exercise 6:
Jade Hop

This is a powerful grounding exercise. Too much thinking, worrying, reading, computers, and other close work causes our energy to stay in our head—we become ungrounded and unstable. We become top heavy and not centered in the hara, which is 2 inches below the belly-button. Life becomes difficult when we have excessive energy in our head. However, when we learn to ground our energy in our hara area, answers to our problems come more easily; we see life as it is. When we are grounded we feel more relaxed and able to calmly handle any situation life brings to us.

1. Stand and simply start hopping up and down, 1 or 2 inches, in a relaxed manner. You can also use a jump rope for variety.
2. Continue until you feel slightly winded, 1 or 2 minutes.

This simple but potent exercise strengthens the sexual organs and stimulates the pituitary gland in the mid-brain and the thymus gland over the heart. It builds strength in the legs and rejuvenates the kidneys and adrenal glands. It also helps to prevent the formation of kidney stones. The Jade Hop decongests the head, sinuses, and lungs to allow fresh blood to circulate in the head and eyes for better vision. It also enhances circulation in the lymphatic system to detoxify the body and build immunity.

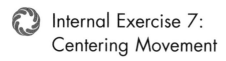 Internal Exercise 7:
Centering Movement

After grounding—moving your energy down and away from your head—centering your energy is next. Centering your body places you in harmony with life, which helps you to see the correct answers to your problems. This wonderful movement loosens the back and squeezes the internal organs.

1. Stand with your feet shoulder-width apart and relax. Bend your knees slightly; let your arms hang loosely like ropes, while your mid-body and shoulders move. Let your breathing be natural.
2. Move your right shoulder forward and up in a circle, and then lower it backward.
3. Do the same with the left shoulder, moving it forward, up in a circle, and back.
4. As your left shoulder is moving upward and back, let your right shoulder come forward and up again. Alternate in this manner while twisting your waist with the rotating movement.
5. When you first begin, perform easy, small circles; gradually increase to larger circles.

Do not tighten up while performing this exercise: You must relax! Become like a rag doll. Just hang loose! Put a smile on your face and pretend you are doing a dance.

The Centering Movement helps to expel toxins from the body, absorbs fresh chi, increases your vitality, and heals the internal organs. While twisting and squeezing your internal organs, it massages them thoroughly. It helps to release gas, so belching and rumbling sounds are a sign of toxins being expelled from the body. It is also great for weight reduction, eases shoulder and back pain, and strengthens the sexual organs. It helps to drain and massage the lymphatic glands. At first, perform 16 times. Eventually, perform for 3 minutes non-stop.

HEALING SOUNDS FOR THE LIVER AND KIDNEY SYSTEMS

The practice of the Healing Sounds taught by the Universal Tao will also improve your vision by working on the two vital organ systems that are the root of your vision, the liver system and the kidney system.

 ### The Liver's Healing Sound

Associated organ: Gallbladder
Element: Wood
Season: Spring
Negative emotions: Anger, aggression
Positive emotions: Kindness, self-expansion, identity
Sound: Sh-h-h-h-h-h-h
Parts of the body: Inner legs, groin, diaphragm, ribs
Senses: Sight, tears, eyes
Taste: Sour
Color: Green

1. Become aware of the liver, and feel the connection between the eyes and the liver (fig. 5.4).

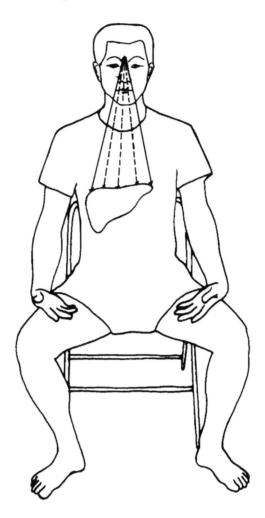

Fig. 5.4. Become aware of the liver.

2. Place your arms at your sides, palms out. Take a deep breath as you slowly swing your arms up and over your head. Follow with the eyes (fig. 5.5).

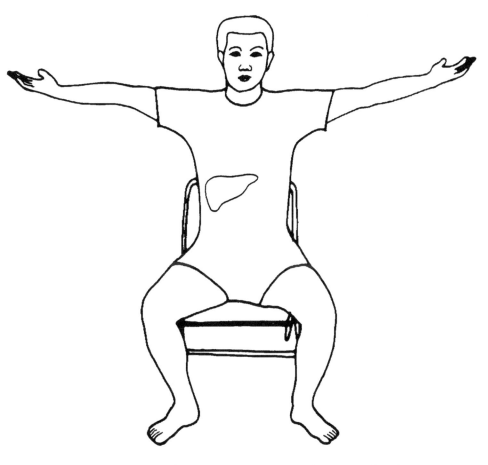

Fig. 5.5. Slowly swing your arms up and over your hand.

3. Interlace the fingers and rotate the palms to face the ceiling (see fig. 5.6 on page 86). Push out at the heels of the palms (see fig. 5.7 on page 87) and feel the stretch through the arms and into the shoulders. Bend slightly to the left, exerting a gentle pull on the liver (see fig. 5.8 on page 87).

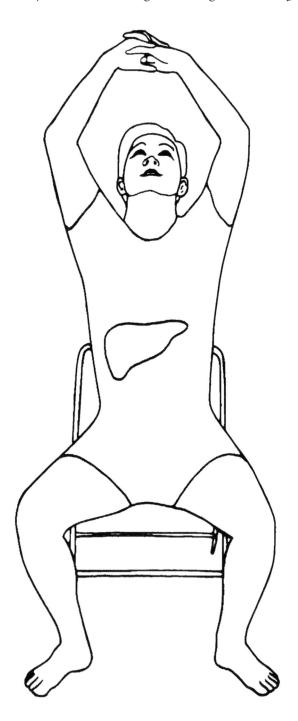

Fig. 5.6. Interlace the fingers and rotate the palms.

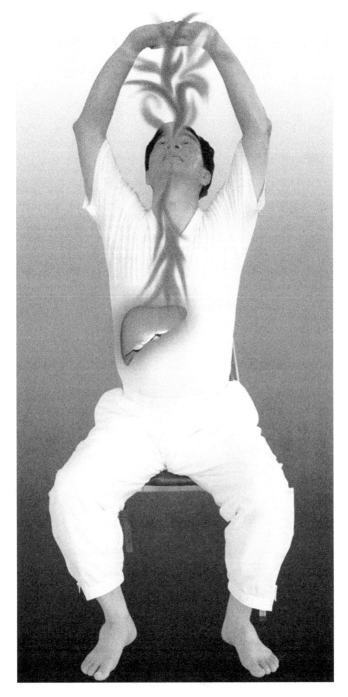

Fig. 5.7. Push out at the heels of the palms, pushing more
with the right arm.

4. Exhale on the sound sh-h-h-h-h-h-h (fig. 5.8), sub-vocally. Envision and feel that a sac encloses the liver and is compressing and expelling the excess heat and anger (fig. 5.9).

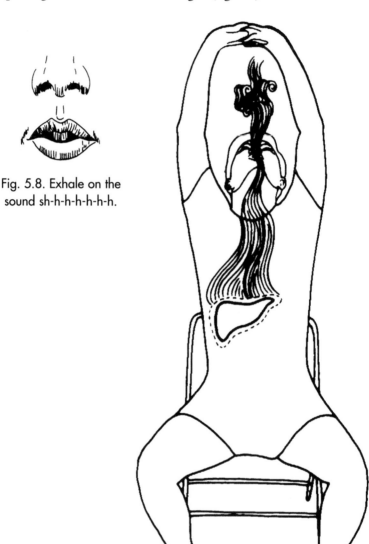

Fig. 5.8. Exhale on the sound sh-h-h-h-h-h-h.

Fig. 5.9. Feel that a sac encloses the liver and is compressing.

5. When you have exhaled completely, unlock the fingers, and pressing out with the heels of the palms (fig. 5.10), breathe into the liver slowly; imagine a bright green color with the quality of kindness entering the liver. Gently bring the arms back to the side by lowering the shoulders. Place your hands on your lap, palms up, and rest.

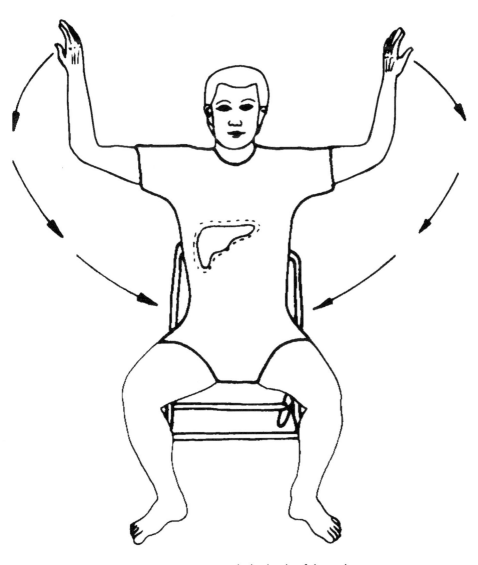

Fig. 5.10. Press out with the heels of the palms.

6. Close the eyes, breathe normally, smile down to the liver and imagine you're still making the sound (fig. 5.11). Be aware of sensations. Sense the energy exchange.

7. Do this 3 to 6 times. For anger, red and watery eyes, or a sour or bitter taste, and for detoxifying the liver, repeat 9 to 36 times.

A Taoist axiom about controlling anger says: "If you've done the liver sound 30 times and you are still angry at someone, you have the right to slap that person."

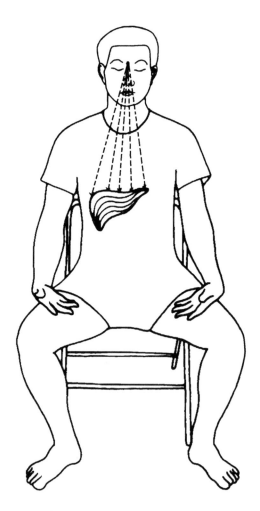

Fig. 5.11. Close your eyes and smile down to the liver.

The Kidneys' Healing Sound

Associated organ: Bladder

Element: Water

Season: Winter

Negative emotion: Fear

Positive emotions: Gentleness, alertness, stillness

Sound: Choo-oo-oo-oo

Parts of the body: Side of foot, inner leg, chest

Senses: Hearing, ears, bones

Taste: Salty

Color: Black or dark blue

1. Become aware of the kidneys (fig. 5.12).

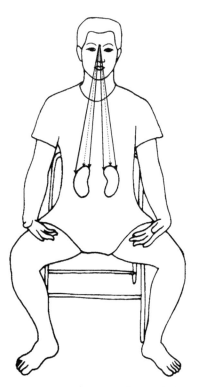

Fig. 5.12. Become aware of your kidneys.

2. Place the legs together, ankles and knees touching. Take a deep breath as you bend forward and hook your hands around your knees; with hands clasped and arms straight, pull back on your arms. Feel the pull at the back where the kidneys are; look up, and tilt the head back without straining (fig. 5.13).

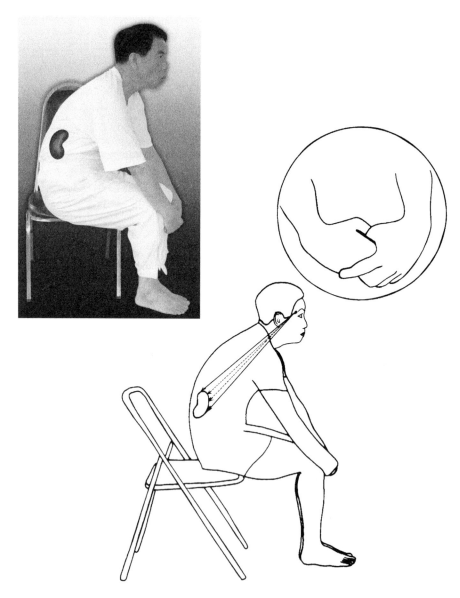

Fig. 5.13. Hook the hands around the knees.

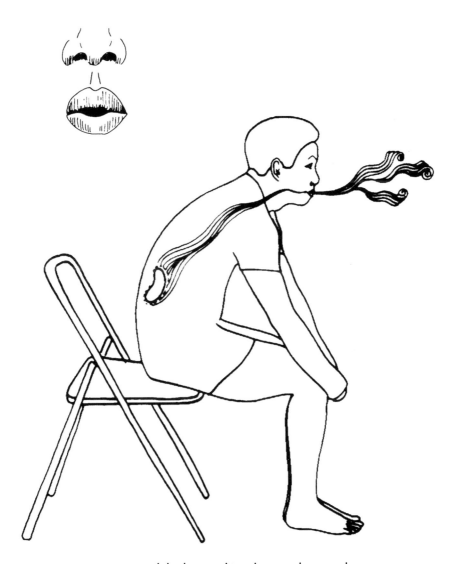

Fig. 5.14. Round the lips, making the sound one makes
when blowing out a candle.

3. Round the lips and silently make the sound one makes in blowing
   out a candle (fig. 5.14). At the same time, press the middle abdomen, between the sternum and navel, toward the spine. Imagine
   the excess heat; wet, sick energy; and fear being squeezed out from
   the membrane around the kidneys (see fig. 5.15 on page 94).

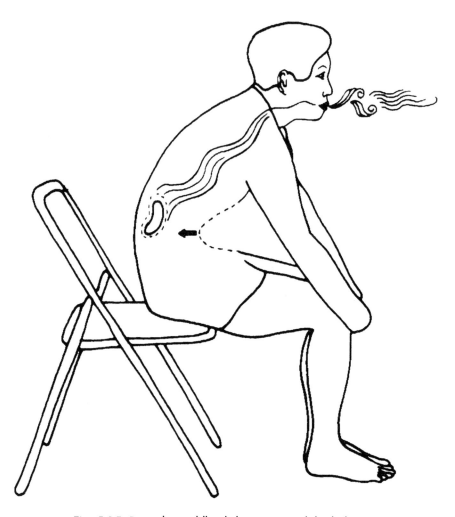

Fig. 5.15. Press the middle abdomen toward the kidneys.

4. When you have exhaled completely, sit up and slowly breathe into the kidneys, imagining a bright blue energy with the quality of gentleness entering the kidneys. Separate the legs so they are in line with your hips and rest your hands, palms up, on your thighs (fig. 5.16).

5. Close the eyes and breathe normally. Smile to the kidneys, as you imagine that you are still making the sound. Pay attention to sensations. Be aware of the exchange of energy around the kidneys, hands, head, and legs.

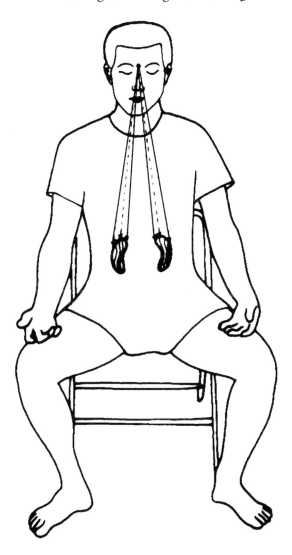

Fig. 5.16. Close your eyes and smile down to the kidneys.

6. When your breathing calms down, repeat 3 to 6 times.
7. For back pain, fatigue, dizziness, ringing in the ears, or detoxifying the kidneys, repeat 9 to 36 times.

Special Oriental Do-In

Self-Healing Massage Techniques for Healthy Eyesight

DO-IN CLEARS BLOCKAGES FOR EYE AND BRAIN HEALING

From the Orient have come stories of miraculous healing powers never before seen in the West. What do the Orientals know that the West has yet to learn? One of their great secrets is a self-massage practice called Do-In. The Chinese refer to self-massage practice as self-acupressure or working the meridian pressure points for the internal organs. Many of the Japanese and Chinese sages who practice and teach Do-In in Japan are reported to be well over a hundred years young and going strong!

The basic purpose of Do-In self-healing massage is to break up blockages in the organs, meridians, nerves, muscles, and tendons, which increases blood and chi or energy circulation throughout the entire body. When these conditions are met, the body and eyes automatically receive healing energy. Frances B., a dear friend of ours from Toronto, was suffering from partial paralysis of her left arm. After a few days of performing Do-In and Chi Kung exercise she was able to move her arm freely and without any pain.

Some of the most vital areas to massage are the neck and solar plexus (also referred to as the hara or belly). The neck, according to Chi Kung masters, is not only the gateway between the mental and the physical centers, but is also a gateway to the emotional and spiritual centers in the body. A verse in the Bible says: "This wicked and stiff-necked generation . . ." and then describes the terrible things that are going to happen to them. We actually see with our brain, through the eyes. That is why circulation to the brain is so important for vision. Mikhael Aivanhov, a Bulgarian yogi master states, "The brain and the solar plexus work together. If there is a blockage in the neck and the communication is not very good, you must massage the neck in the region of the cervical vertebrae so as to reestablish the current going from the solar plexus to the brain." This is also important to allow nerve and blood circulation to flow to the tiny nerves and capillaries in the eyes and eye muscles.

Do-In has many varied techniques and modalities for self-healing. When you improve circulation to one part of the body, the healing benefits are felt in other parts of the body also. The following is a very simple Do-In routine. Each area should be rubbed firmly 9 to 12 times, following the order given below. The head and neck should be massaged with the fingers. Rub the arms, legs, and trunk with the palms of your hands. Massage your feet with your fingers.

Daily Do-In Self-Healing Massage Routine

- Rub the crown of the head and temples for mental clarity.
- Rub the ears to heat up the body and invigorate the kidneys.
- Rub the eyes to regenerate the liver, improve vision, and freshen the spirit.
- Rub the nose to help heal heart problems.
- Rub the mouth to help improve stomach digestion.

- Rub the nostrils and cheeks to eliminate mucus and sinus problems and to cleanse the lungs.
- Rub the neck for emotional problems, stress, and to increase vitality; also enhances calmness and poise.
- Rub the arms for heart problems, nervousness, and emotional love problems.
- Rub the chest and upper back for depression, grief, and the courage to face life without fear.
- Rub the heart area for greater circulation and spiritual love.
- Rub the liver (under right rib cage), to strengthen the eyesight and for sustaining energy.
- Rub the kidneys for better hearing or ear problems.
- Rub the big toe to clear the brain and achieve mental clarity.
- Rub the four small toes to help heal the eyesight and hearing.
- Rub the feet for mental and physical grounding and physical strength.
- Rub your legs to release past problems and to place your mind in the present moment.
- Rub your buttocks for sciatic nerve problems, tension, or stress.
- Rub the sacrum for lower back pain, hemorrhoids, and menstrual cramps.
- Rub your belly (hara) for abundant health and centering, and to gain wisdom, intuition, and insight.
- Rub in the exact order as outlined above for grounding and centering.

Do not massage the head, ears, or eye areas at night, because the energy may go to the head and keep you awake. Perform Do-In head massage in the morning. Always finish a Do-In massage session with a belly massage. This brings the energy to the center of the body, where it creates balance, centeredness, and calmness.

Jean Rofidal, writing in *DO-IN: Eastern Massage and Yoga Techniques*, says, "Many people think they can get by without paying any respect to the rules of the Universal Order which may be classified under four main headings: nourishment, respiration, exercise, and meditation. . . ." However, "they give us the opportunity of doing something about our well being. For instance, by acting on the exterior of our bodies, we can act on the interior and by acting on the gross, we act on the subtle. . . . Do-In affords a splendid method of acting on our bodies physically, mentally, and spiritually."

HEART AND BELLY

When the ancients talked about the heart, they were talking about the belly or hara. "When initiates speak of the intelligence of the heart," according to Master Aivanhov, "no one, not even the theologians, has understood why it is the heart which possesses the veritable intelligence, nor what this intelligence is. To the initiates, the heart is not the pump which propels the blood through the organism, but it is another heart, the solar plexus (hara or belly area)."

The brain and the mind can never have true or correct answers for us, as they are merely intellectual surface tools for everyday life. The head or brain-mind thinking most always gets us in trouble. That is why Zen, yoga, and Taoist masters tell their students to "cut off your head"—figuratively, of course! They teach us to stop worrying or constantly thinking about our problems. Instead, we need to concentrate and breathe into the lower belly, or hara, the center of our being (God/Tao center), for peace, guidance, health, and happiness.

Do-In is practiced to prevent disease, maintain a high-level of health, and to cultivate our individual chi. Do-In practitioners also use hara massage to help cure illnesses. Ayurveda and Chinese medicine both concur that disease begins in the hara or belly area (stomach, intestines, liver). Ayurvedic medicine says: "There is no disease without first gastrointestinal derangement." Chinese medicine refers to the hara as "central energy," meaning it is where health and energy are generated and maintained. And when the colon, stomach, and liver are functioning below par, showing up as weak digestion, fatigue, constipation, diarrhea, hepatitis, diabetes, low blood sugar, and so on, the eyesight also weakens and becomes diseased.

Oriental medicine teaches that we must open the blockages in the physical body to receive energy and healing. Several years ago Robert Zuraw developed an energy imbalance and illness due to Agent Orange poisoning in Vietnam, and to eating too much dairy. He began performing hara massage and overcame his mysterious illness. His vision also improved every year. There is no limit to how well we can see. With the proper knowledge, understanding, and practice, you too can have good vision for as long as you live. This is really good news. But you have to take action to follow through on these valuable vision and health training secrets.

BALANCING UPPER AND LOWER BODY CENTERS

We use our brain machine far too much, to our own detriment, unlike our ancient ancestors, who had slower brain activity, no technology, less worry and anxiety, and less intellectual thinking. Excessive thinking and negative emotions move our energy up to the head, instead of down in the hara or belly area, where it needs to be to stay calm. This area is also called the second brain, as it is where we get our "gut" feelings or intuition.

Most of us refuse to see that we caused our own problems in the first place, by making emotional or irrational decisions. Traditional Chinese Medicine (TCM) talks about those who suffer from an *excess* of the seven human emotions—joy, anger, anxiety, worry, grief, apprehension, and fear. These emotions, in excess, are the cause of much depression and emotional diseases. We have an epidemic of such mental illnesses and emotional problems in the world today, which can be a direct cause of poor health and faulty vision.

Taoists call these mental problems "sentimental diseases." Sentimental diseases are caused by the misuse or abuse of negative emotions. For example, people die of an excess of grief; hair can turn white overnight from an excess of fear or stress; losing a job or a break-up of a relationship has caused many to stay depressed for years, also causing headaches, bulimia, anorexia, and crying spells. Worry causes spleen and stomach illness and poor digestion. Diarrhea or a weak bladder can be caused by fright. Heart attacks have happened after "winning" at the racetrack. Anxiety and fear have kept many from success, with paralyzing effect. Excess anger can cause strokes, liver problems, and weak vision. These are examples of "sentimental diseases."

Because we overuse our brains, we are more strongly afflicted with the seven negative sentimental emotions. As a result we suffer from an excess of energy in the upper body, and a deficiency in the lower body, especially the hara or belly area. By reversing this energy pattern, we can restore our balance between the yin (lower part of the body) and the yang (upper part of the body) to increase our health and vision. We can balance our head with our hara and overcome imbalanced negative mental states by making healthy food choices and performing Hara Massage and Foot Slapping daily.

HARA MASSAGE FOR UNLIMITED ENERGY

Hara Massage is for everyone. It is easy and fun to do. It takes about ten minutes to perform before going to sleep or you can do it in the morning before getting out of bed. After a few minutes of "belly rubbing" you will feel more energy, along with less stress and nervous exhaustion. Your vision will also improve more quickly if you perform Hara Massage daily. Start today on your road to energy and vitality.

Healing Hara Massage

There are three power centers in the abdomen:

1. The solar plexus, in the pit of the abdomen (arch of the rib cage)

2. Behind the bellybutton area

3. The lower tan tien, 1½ inches below the bellybutton

We learned these deep Hara Massage techniques from Chinese and Japanese Do-In and Chi Kung masters. They recommend massaging the entire hara (stomach, liver, and intestines), from under the rib cage to the pubic bone. Massage deep and slow, with your fingers, knuckles, and fist. Massage the entire abdominal area just before bedtime, and again before getting out of bed in the morning. When the hara is relaxed during sleep, the internal organs and eyesight are allowed to heal naturally. Plus, it opens us up to receive the proper spiritual guidance or intuition for the next day's activity.

Massage the entire abdomen for a few minutes daily, and you will experience peace, tranquility, self-control, and answers to your problems. It is also a good idea to receive a 30- to 60-minute Hara Massage from a massage therapist. In Japan, a Hara Massage therapist works on the entire abdomen for an hour or more. Many people experience healing after these intense Hara Massage sessions.

FOOT SLAPPING TO INVIGORATE THE KIDNEYS AND NOURISH THE EYES AND LIVER

Foot Slapping Balances Water and Fire in the Body

For good health, the body requires water to move upward and fire downward. This is because the head and brain must remain cool and calm, while the hands and feet remain warm. When one is ill, the head is usually hot with fire, and the hands and feet are cool, cold, or clammy and moist.

Slapping the bottom of the feet brings the fire down and helps the water go up. When the Kidney point (Yongquan) on the sole of each foot is opened, you will be able to draw the energy of the earth into your body (earth magnetism). Slapping the Yongquan point can also help those who have performed Chi Kung incorrectly or who have had an energy blockage (chi not flowing smoothly throughout the body), constant nausea, headaches, dizziness, hot head, cold hands, ear ringing, and so on.

Foot Slapping harmonizes the heart and kidneys. When the kidneys become healthy and vigorous, they nourish the liver, which also enhances the eyesight for near and far vision.

Positive Benefits of Foot Slapping or Tapping

Chi Kung Master Huang Runtian, writing in *Treasured Qigong of Traditional Medical School*, states that Foot Slapping or Tapping "can nourish the liver and improve eyesight; curing chronic diseases of the liver, gallbladder and eyesight diseases (near-sightedness, far-sightedness, and poor-sightedness)." He continues: "As a result of conscientious practicing of the Qigong exercise, the liver-wood nourished by sufficient kidney-water and abundant 'earth Qi' would be full of vigor and vitality. Thus, the Qigong can nourish the liver and make the eyes clear."

Chinese medicine claims that the following ailments are helped by Foot Tapping or Slapping: yin (cold) deficiency, yang (hot) excess, upper body heat excess, lower body deficiency (ungroundedness), kidney and heart problems, excessive rise of liver yang, seminal emissions, night sweats, heart palpitations, poor memory, insomnia, mental stress, neurasthenia, migraine headaches, knee and back pain, blood deficiency, burning red face, mental depression, poor eyesight, liver and gallbladder problems.

"In practicing Dao-Yin [Do-In], you need not believe in it, but you must do the exercise earnestly. You will get benefits from it, whether you believe it or not," says Master Runtian.

Personal Experience of Foot Slapping

While visiting Zen Taoist master Hyunoong Sunim in Washington State, I (Robert Lewanski) was awakened early one morning by a loud clapping sound. I found out later that he was slapping his feet three hundred times. When he came to Royal Oak, Michigan, for a seminar a few years later, I tested his eyesight, and found that he had better than 20–20 vision. His vision was in the range of 40–10, about three times better than 20–20 normal vision! He could read the ten-foot Snellen Eye Chart at forty feet away without glasses or contacts—a super feat for someone in his early forties!

The Do-In Foot Slapping Technique for Strengthening the Kidneys and Adjusting Energy Levels

The regular practice of this Do-In Foot Slapping technique has proven to renew physical and mental health, restore good vision, and promote long life.

The goal of Foot Slapping—in which the sole of the foot is slapped with the open palm—is to open up two energy points: the Kidney acupuncture point, Yongquan, on the foot, and the Laogong acupuncture point on the palm (fig. 6.1).

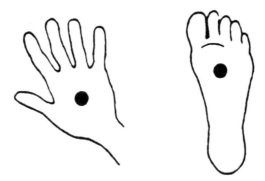

Fig. 6.1. The Laogong point in the palm of the hand and the Yongquan point on the sole of the foot

1. Sit on a chair, close your eyes, and relax your body.
2. Breathe naturally. Rid your mind of distractions. Be silent for a few minutes.

3. Open your eyes. Place your right foot on your left knee.

4. With the open palm of your left hand, slap the arch of your right foot, so that the Laogong acupoint in the middle of the left hand slaps on the Yongquan acupoint on your right foot.

5. Just relax your palm, and hit with an even force—not too hard, but medium. Do not slap your foot with a stiff or rigid hand; keep your palm cupped and your wrist area loose. Slap at an even slow tempo, about 1 second for each slap.

6. Place your left foot on your right knee and slap it with your right palm in the same manner.

7. Meditate or be silent for a few minutes.

Begin by slapping each foot 50 times each morning and night; over time work up to 100 and later 200. Once the points are opened—over several weeks of practice—foot slapping 50 times before bed will be sufficient.

Caution: If you are a beginner at Foot Slapping, slap your foot gently for the first 2 weeks. Do not cause yourself pain or soreness. Take it easy and relax into it. Increase the force as you improve. Once the acupoint is opened, the sting, soreness, or redness will no longer be there.

If you have low blood pressure or hypoglycemia, place one hand on the top of your head while the other hand slaps your foot. Do not practice Foot Slapping if you suffer from a serious health problem, such as cancer or a heart condition, or are extremely weak. If you are seriously ill, just rub the foot and finish by rubbing the belly a few minutes.

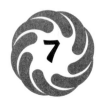

Nutritional Secrets for Visual Clarity

RESTORING YOUR HEALTH AND EYESIGHT WITH WHOLE FOODS

Good nutrition is vitally important in your quest for strong and healthy eye muscles, nerves, and blood vessels. These eye components determine the health and vitality of our vision. If you are weak, tired, or run down, with dull unclear vision, the immediate cause is malnutrition or malabsorption of vital food nutrients.

Health and nutrition is our own personal responsibility. How we eat determines our state of health. If we eat devitalized foods, we develop a devitalized body, and our eyes become dim and lifeless. Hippocrates, the father of modern medicine, once stated, "Your food should be your medicine, and your medicine should be your food."

Food is our direct link to Mother Earth. Natural food gives us natural chemical elements such as minerals, vitamins, enzymes, and fiber. These are the life-giving elements that feed our cells, tissues, hair, skin, bones, teeth, and eyes. Without a daily flow of these powerful little dynamos in your system, you can forget about good health and perfect eyesight!

Make nutrition, health, and fitness your daily routine and habit. Health should be your first and foremost hobby. Is a car, house, boat, or other expensive "toy" more important than the health of your most important possessions—your self and your loved ones?

You have probably heard the sentiment, "Physician, heal thyself." Who is this physician? You are! If you seek good health and perfect eyesight, only you can give yourself the necessary understanding to apply the laws of nutrition to your divine temple. Only you can know how to flow with the natural rhythm of life—when you are hungry, tired, sleepy, thirsty, and so on. Only you can decide to eat when you have true hunger, rest when tired, sleep when sleepy, drink when thirsty, exercise when full of energy, eliminate when nature calls, and meditate when the spirit moves you. When you pay attention to your original nature—your internal physiological needs and intuitive feelings—you will be led to a natural moderation in all your activities.

The eyes are the most abused organs of the body. They reflect the condition of the body organs, especially the liver and gallbladder, which work together to detox the body of excess chemicals, fats, junk food, and environmental poisons. If you have a weak, malfunctioning liver and gallbladder, your eyes may show some of the following symptoms and characteristics: aching, jaundice, bulging, bloodshot, watery, spots, and itching.

The Oriental sages assure us that in addition to Do-In and Chi Kung health and energy cultivation exercises, meditation, and prayer, wholesome nutrition—consisting mainly of whole natural foods, such as vegetables, fruits, seeds, grains, herbs, and herbal teas—is key to maintaining super health and overcoming illness. Learn to eat correctly, and your vision and energy will zoom with rocketlike power.

FIVE HEALTHY NUTRITION KEYS
TO PERFECT EYESIGHT

Health Key Number 1:
Eat Only when Hungry and
Take Liquids Only when Thirsty

It is said that "very few people die from starvation, but millions die prematurely from overeating." Another wise jokester stated: "Half the food we eat feeds us, the other half feeds the doctor." Overeating leads to malnutrition and poor eyesight.

Our stomach, which houses the digestive system, operates like a potbelly stove. Overstuff the stove with wood, and you will get nothing but smoke; it will refuse to burn smoothly. But fill the same stove three-quarters full and the wood will burn beautifully. Your stomach will also not burn (digest) food smoothly if you stuff it with food. Eat until you are three-quarters full and stop! Health and energy will be there for those who heed this advice.

Overeating destroys the nutritional value of the food eaten, whether it is from a single meal or from eating too soon after a previous meal. Even whole, natural food will not digest properly if you stuff your "stove." Putting more food in before the previously ingested food is completely digested always results in putrefaction and fermentation. They in turn cause indigestion and toxemia.

Indigestion is one of the greatest causes of energy loss, disease, and poor eyesight. The immune system is directly connected to the power and efficiency of good digestion, assimilation, absorption, and elimination of food. There is a saying "Eat to live—not live to eat." Many people live only to see how much they can stuff down their gullet. They live only for "mouth amusement," or to tickle their taste buds. Food must be delicious, nutritious, and tasteful, but don't obsess over it. If you eat wholesome, nutritious foods, you will be satisfied on less food—and be better nourished. If food is digested and assimilated well—with no stomachaches, indigestion, or gas—the eyes receive a good flow of micronutrients and you will experience better results while performing your eye exercises.

There is an inner physiological voice within you that tells you when, what, and how much you need to eat every day. Listen to your body intelligence. What do you feel? Are you really hungry? Or do you eat out of boredom, depression, or emotions?

Positive Sign of True Hunger: If you are truly hungry, you will be happy, joyous, with a real yearning for food at mealtimes. What are the physical and psychological signs of hunger? Your mouth should water. The tongue is the upper gateway to the lower gastrointestinal system. It should be pink and clear, with no white, yellow, green, brown, or black coatings, which indicate that undigested food has not evacuated the stomach, small intestines, or colon. Hunger is properly indicated by mouth and throat sensations—not by stomach pangs or grumbling, which indicate toxins or undigested food in the stomach. Such symptoms also indicate overindulgence in excessively stimulating foods and drinks such as meat, dairy products, processed foods, sugar, candy, cake, soda, other commercial junk food, and alcohol.

Your energy should also be high before eating. It is not a good time to eat when you are experiencing tiredness, fatigue, emotional upsets, or stress. Rest thirty to sixty minutes first, then eat when your energy is restored. Food digests smoothly and completely when you are rested and full of energy and vitality.

Important Health Note: Eat only when hungry. As a Taoist proverb says, "When you know when enough is enough, you will always have enough."

Health Key Number 2: Chew Your Food Well— Your Key to Good Eyesight and Health

Observe the noon lunch hour at an office. The robot-like workers rush from their desks to the nearest "fast-food greasy-spoon slop-house." They gulp and swallow their food like swilling swine. Lifeless junk food is then washed down with a large sugared soda, coffee, or tea. These people feel that they must eat fast because there is so much work to do. They rush back to work. Then they are exhausted and stressed out by three or four o'clock, when they reach for another coffee and donut to boost their sagging spirits. Fast foods lead to fast diseases and a fast trip to the cemetery.

This scenario goes on every day in every big city in the world. And the hospitals and morgues are filled with such sad souls that didn't have time to chew, relax, digest, assimilate, meditate, and contemplate on where the food came from, where they are going on this mud-ball, and what life is all about.

Food gulped down on the run cannot possibly be digested properly. Proper chewing gets our digestive juices flowing. It gets the food ready for thorough assimilation in the gastrointestinal tract and healthy bowel elimination. Bowel problems start with poor eating habits. Eating too fast prevents good digestion; consequently, the food sits in the stomach and putrefies. As a result, "gas wars" are going on in millions of workplaces. We have no real gas shortage! Scientists should find a way to hook up that gas to power our cities!

It all gets back to the art of chewing. Our stomach has no teeth to handle unchewed food. Although we did hear of a man who swallowed his false teeth so he could gulp his food and chew later! Seriously, digestion starts with the saliva in the mouth. The enzyme ptyalin in saliva breaks down starch in the mouth before it enters the stomach for further digestion.

We bypass the first step of digestion when we gulp and run. Long-lived people always chew their food slowly—twenty to thirty times per mouthful. Macrobiotics say: "Chew fine, think fine. Chew rough, think rough." Think about that.

Enjoy the taste of your food; this makes your digestive juices flow smoothly, and enables you to utilize the essential nutritional ingredients of the food for improved eyesight.

Health Key Number 3:
Eat Mostly Whole, Natural Foods in
Season, and in Your Climate

The optimum diet for perfect eyesight, health, and longevity is one that includes plenty of whole grains (rice, barley, millet, rye, wheat, oats, buckwheat, spelt, amaranth, kamut, and pasta made from them) and vegetables (lightly steamed in winter and raw in summer).

Supplement this basic whole foods diet with some raw fruits eaten mostly in warm summer months. Nuts and seeds (almonds, walnuts, cashews, sesame seeds, sunflower and pumpkin seeds) and beans (green and yellow split peas, adzuki, navy, kidney, black, garbanzo, lentils, lima) should be soaked in water overnight to revive their life force, or used in soups and cooking. If you are not a vegetarian, eat only small amounts of animal foods to maintain good health.

Fish from Alaska, Australia, or New Zealand is virtually free of mercury and harmful chemicals. All other types of fish from large coastal cities are highly contaminated. Organic chicken and turkey are better than commercial brands. Organic eggs and milk far surpass commercial variety in quality and nutrients.

If you want to feel and look your best, consume foods that are grown within a 500-mile radius of where you live, and eat them in their proper season. That means eat seasonal fruits and vegetables when they are harvested in your area. For example, in Michigan, asparagus is ready in May, early leafy greens in June, berries in June and July, melons and corn in August and September, apples in September and October, and so on.

Tender fresh raw fruits and vegetables are ready to eat in the spring and summer for a reason. They cleanse the liver of toxins that accumulate during the winter months. Cherries and berries, especially blueberries, blackberries, strawberries, and raspberries, help to detox the liver, cleanse the blood, and increase iron and oxygen in the system.

Cooked grains, beans, soups, pasta, and steamed root vegetables are more suitable for cold winter months. They impart strength and maintain heat in the body, hands, and feet. Raw food is loaded with potassium—a cooling mineral that cools the blood and body during hot summer months. Cooked whole foods, on the other hand, are higher in sodium, phosphorus, nitrogen—warming minerals that warm up the blood and body in cold winter months.

If you listen to your intuition (body intelligence), it will lead you to the right foods for the right climate and season. Stay away from extreme one-sided diets. They only cause poor health and weak eyesight.

Health Key Number 4: Super Nutrient-Rich Foods for Perfect Eyesight

Seeds

Seeds such as pumpkin seeds and sunflower seeds contain the life-giving force of nature bundled up in a tiny package. Seeds are the beginning of another life. They come from life and they give us life when we eat them.

Sunflower seeds are a supreme food for the eyes. They contain vitamin B_2, which helps to prevent and overcome photophobia. They are also high in vitamin D, the sunshine vitamin. The sunflower seed plant turns its head to the sun, thereby absorbing the glorious life-giving light. Eat a tablespoon of sunflower seeds daily in your cereal or after soaking them overnight and notice how you can easily endure sunlight or headlight glare.

Carrots

Carrots and carrot juice work wonders for night vision. Carrots are high in vitamin A. The body does not require a high intake of vitamin A daily, because it is stored in the liver for future use. So, a six-ounce glass of carrot juice or five carrots a week is enough to give you plenty of beta-carotene and vitamin A for sparkling clear vision.

Edgar Cayce, the "Sleeping Prophet," speaks highly of carrots as a remedy for many ailments in his dietary remedy books.

We recommend eating only organic carrots. Carrots are noted for soaking up whatever is in the soil. Commercial carrots are packed full of health-destroying chemical fertilizers, pesticides, and the latest kinds of devastating immune-system-destroying chemical sprays. Unlike these commercial varieties, organic carrots are naturally sweet and delicious. They are loaded with over four times the vitamins, minerals, trace elements, and healing power as the anemic chemical types.

Our gracious Mother Earth will have the last word on this! She may be getting ready to rumble and shake up the sleeping mechanical robots who are choking her life-roots. Eat organic vegetables and be on the safe side. She will place you in her protective arms if you follow her natural laws of food and health.

Healing Herbs

Blueberry, bilberry, and raspberry herb teas are all good for night vision. Parsley contains vitamin B_2, which helps to improve day vision. Eyebright herb tea has been used for centuries for improving the eyesight. Steep a teaspoon of eyebright in a cup of hot water for twenty minutes; drink a cup a day. Dandelion root tea improves distant vision (nearsightedness). Dandelion leaf tea helps you to see better close (farsightedness).

Teas made from Chinese litchi berries and chrysanthemum flowers are highly acclaimed in the Orient for promoting better vision and reducing liver toxicity. Use the Chinese herbs for a month, then change to the Western herbs (eyebright and dandelion) the following month.

Licorice root is an excellent herb to reduce inflammation and mucus and to improve vision. Licorice is also said to enhance memory and mental clarity. Use no more than a quarter teaspoon of licorice powder in water daily. Or chew on a small piece of licorice stick. Ayurvedic physician Dr. Vinod Verma recommends: "Take [licorice] as a preventive measure after age 35, as many people tend to get problems with their vision around that age."

Foods that Heal, Cleanse, and Strengthen the Liver and Eyes

The following vegetables, fruits, and seeds will strengthen and heal your liver, eyes, and immune system: yams, squash, potatoes, tomatoes, carrots, beets, dandelion greens, celery, cabbage, broccoli, chard, kale, collards, green beans, fresh snow peas and green peas, olives, radishes, mushrooms, celery, grapes, blueberries, raspberries, plums, prunes, litchi berries, mango, grapefruit, lemons, limes, sunflower seeds, pumpkin seeds, umeboshi plums, and pickles. Also, include all the other vegetables in your diet for variety.

Green vegetables help to clear the eyes and prevent eye inflammation. Whole grains contain vitamin B-complex, which strengthens eye nerves and the entire nervous system. Buckwheat contains rutin to repair and heal cells and tissues. Barley helps to heal tumors and inflammations. Oatmeal is rich in silicon for sparkling eyes, lustrous hair, and strong nails. Supplement with kombucha tea, miso, apple cider vinegar, blue green algae, green kamut, spirulina, and green barley magma. Other herbs that help to clear away liver toxicity and improve eyesight are rose hips, bupleurum, haritaki, and amalaki.

Health Key Number 5: Avoid Toxic Foods that Cause Ill Health and Vision Problems

Did you know that the "average American diet" is costing us over 900 billion dollars yearly in medical bills? The average American is annually consuming 150 pounds of refined white sugar, 85 pounds of processed oils and fats, 150 pounds of white flour, 15 pounds of white rice, cases of alcohol, and thousands of cigarettes! By comparison, in the early 1900s, Americans ate only 5 pounds of white sugar per person. In the early 1900s only 6 percent of the population was nearsighted. Today, 75 percent of the population suffers from poor health and poor vision; they require eyeglasses and eventually eye surgery!

As a nation, we should be ashamed of ourselves. Disease is on the rise. Hospitals are filled to capacity. Jails and mental institutions are overcrowded. These are tragic statistics. They show the power of mass hypnotism via the media—TV, papers, radio—concerning our health or lack thereof. Junk foods, medicines, alcohol, and fast living are all promoted by large corporations, with little regard for our health, sanity, or well-being. Many people are walking around today in a "somnambulistic trance" (as Gurdjieff once said), addicted to material things, power, greed, fast foods, sugared drinks, drugs, coffee, cigarettes, and alcohol! Where it will end, no one knows.

Medical doctors are now finding a close link between dietary habits and disease causation. Holistic doctors have known this for centuries. Good health and good eyesight go hand in hand. Only YOU can take charge of your life, health, and eyesight. Avoid junk foods and poisons such as chemical drug medications, antibiotics, white sugar, sodas, candy, cakes, and so on, white table salt, white refined flour (bread, pastries, etc.), solid fats (such as lard or hydrogenated vegetable oil), cheap (extremely rancid) supermarket vegetable oils, canola oil, soy oil, vegetable margarine (made from hydrogenated oils), high salt foods, and commercial dairy products (which are loaded with growth hormones and antibiotics). Shop at your local health food store for higher quality products. They usually stock organic dairy products. However, read the labels; not everything in a health food store is healthy, low fat, or good fat. Buyer beware!

If you practice these teachings, you will enjoy your life in peace, health, and happiness.

Avoid Sugar

Sugar is clearly the most deadly food for your eyesight! This also includes brown sugar, which is just white sugar with molasses added for coloring. Don't be fooled by this gimmick.

Sugar robs all the bones and teeth of calcium and the all-important

B vitamins. It also destroys the pancreas by using up insulin and causing diabetes, obesity, heart disease, skin diseases, poor memory, kidney and liver disorders, and poor eyesight. Sugar forms a "crystalline lens" on the eyes, causing cataracts; it is the main cause of inflamed eyes.

Dr. Jin Otsuka, a leading Japanese authority on nearsightedness, says, "If you feed sugar to a rabbit, the rabbit becomes myopic [nearsighted]." Eaten in excess, even so-called natural sugars, such as honey, maple syrup, rice syrup, and barley malt, weaken the organs and cause poor vision.

The human body only produces one tablespoon of insulin—which is needed for digestion of sugars—daily. If you consume a large glass of carrot juice or fruit juice, and two tablespoons of honey, you will use up your supply of insulin for the day. If you consume four or five times more than this every day for years, you will create hypoglycemia (low blood sugar) and finally diabetes (no insulin produced in the pancreas).

Simple mathematics! Weaken the organs with excess sugars, fats, refined flour, drugs, alcohol, and so on, and you'll be left with zero health—nothing in the balance. Hormones will dry up and disappear. No hormones, no health. No health, no life—period!

If you want to have zestful energy every day, then you'll have to use only natural sweets like honey and maple syrup, and limit your intake to two or three teaspoons a day—no more. Limit your intake of juices also. Fruit juices are concentrated sugars, extracted from the whole fruit. If you need juice, dilute it half with water. You'll save your organs from overworking.

Excess sweets further weaken the adrenal glands, which give us energy during the day. Eat some fruit, especially in warm summer weather. Fruits are good organ cleansers and contain oxygen and iron for blood-building. Fruit is high in potassium (a cooling mineral), so reduce fruit consumption in cold winter weather. The body doesn't need a lot of potassium in the winter. You can, however, occasionally stew or cook some fruit in cool weather if you are healthy. Just don't overdo it.

Avoid Salt

Excessive salt consumption leads to hardening of the arteries, high blood pressure, obesity, and so on. Hardened arteries cause poor circulation to the eyes and weak vision. Excess salt congests the kidneys and eventually creates edema (waterlogged body). Use kelp or powdered vegetable seasoning instead of common table salt. Or use Celtic salt or Himalayan salt, which contain more minerals.

Avoid White Flour

When mixed with the digestive juices, white flour becomes a paste, like plaster of Paris. We become glued up inside, literally blocked up or constipated, from these "refined foods." Many people walk around with fifteen to twenty pounds of dried fecal matter pasted up against their colon walls. They are not happy campers! You see many such angry people driving down the road giving out middle-finger hand signals to other motorists!

Ayurvedic medicine from India teaches that constipation must be overcome in order to improve the eyesight. Constipation is a direct cause of blurred, dim vision, and many major diseases.

Avoid Soybean Products

Soy is a poisonous weed grown for human and animal consumption. Bugs will not eat soy plants, because they detect poison in the plant. People and animals get sick on the stuff. Hair quickly "falls out" on sheep that graze on soy plants. Animals that eat a lot of soy products live only half their normal age. Dogs, cats, and other household pets fed a steady diet of soy tofu and soy products develop illnesses and live only four to six years.

Balding, eye problems, liver problems, yeast infections, poor digestion, fatigue, and so on are closely linked with the use of soy. Tofu, soy "hot dogs," soy tempeh, and soy burgers all fall into the same disease-causing category. These products all cause premature old age! Dr. Carry Reams found "a link between the soybean, balding, and deterioration in the blood." When I (Robert Lewanski) ate soy products and tofu my eyes and health were below par.

Soy is considered a "negative" or left-spin energy plant, unlike healthy natural foods such as grains, beans, vegetables, fruit, organic dairy, seeds, and nuts, which are considered "positive" or right-spin energy plant foods. Positive energy plant foods do not disrupt or damage health and vitality.

Soy oil, tofu, and other soy products contain a poisonous chemical called "phyto-hema-glutinin" or PHG. It is a large protein molecule that causes the blood to clot or stick together like glue, forming plaques on the arterioles, which clog the capillaries in the eyes, ears, and scalp, causing eye problems, ear infections, and hair loss. Peanuts, which some people cannot digest, contain only a small amount of PHG in comparison to soybeans. Use of these products can speed up mental deterioration in young or old people, ultimately causing Alzheimer's. If you use fat-free or oil-free soy products, the health-destroying effects are greatly reduced.

Soy plants can live on "diseased" soil and air. They take in and store toxins from the environment (chemical-laden dead soils and polluted air). Hard salt fertilizers and poisonous sprays are used to produce the toxic soybean. Unbelievable, but true! In the mid-fifties soybeans were "irradiated" to increase their oil content. Soy oil is an industrial oil, not a food oil!

This is a serious matter. Don't take it lightly. Remember: soy products have to be heavily "doctored" to make them almost tolerable to eat. Soybeans undergo hours and hours of processing, cooking, and preparing to make them ready for market. Soybeans cause weak digestion, gas, and a deranged body chemistry in many vegetarians and sensitive people. Vegetarians must be especially wary of eating soy foods and foods with soy products in them. If you want improved health and vision, use other cultural and traditional foods such as beans, peas, and legumes that are high in protein and fiber, easy to cook, and delicious to eat.

Eaten excessively, soy products weaken the gastrointestinal and immune systems. Liver and kidney function are also greatly impaired.

If you are sick, weak, fatigued, or cancerous, avoid soy and tofu completely. If you have poor digestion, gas, or bloating, forget about soy products altogether.

The net protein utilization (NPU) of soy products is a low 10 to 15 percent, which is far too low to maintain good digestion and overall health. The raw soy protein is almost indigestible. However, "free" amino acid soy proteins have positive right-spin energy and are acceptable to eat, because their negative vibration is neutralized— their oil is removed completely. Bragg's Liquid Aminos is a safe positive amino acid to use in your food or cooking.

Avoid Fats

Excess fats cannot be completely digested, assimilated, and absorbed, which results in higher blood cholesterol and blocked arteries. This slows down the circulation to the eyes, as well as to the heart and other major internal organs. Fats are also implicated in diabetes, obesity, gallbladder stones, and liver disease. The liver and gallbladder metabolize fats. A fatty liver causes many eye disorders such as jaundice, dark spots, yellow eyes, red eyes, blindness, astigmatism, crossed eyes, and poor vision.

You'll feel great if you keep your fat intake to around 5 to 10 percent of your diet. Go easy on these high fat foods: milk, cheese, butter, dairy, oils, meats. Eat them sparingly and they will spare your life.

Avoid Dangerous Oils

If you desire good vision and super health avoid, like the plague, all of the following oils and foods containing them: cottonseed, corn, safflower, soy, and canola. Soy and canola oils especially are extremely toxic in the human body! Use these oils to grease your car only! Like soy, canola has negative left-spin energy. Soy and canola oil products weaken the immune system's T cells, weakening the nervous and hormonal systems. These products are systemic toxins, accumulating slowly, causing many disease conditions. PHG in soy and canola kills small rodents fast.

Also avoid oils that deteriorate and become rancid quickly, such as almond, corn, safflower, avocado, and peanut oils. Peanut butter is also loaded with PHG, and will make your blood clot and become gluey. Beware of these oils in many snacks, chips, health candies, and so on.

All margarine is hydrogenated and solid at room temperature, which makes it saturated. Oils are boiled at extremely high temperatures; then a nickel alloy is used as a catalyst to make them hard at room temperature on your dinner table! Margarine will harden your arteries in a jiffy, and cut your life in half. We call it "plastic fat." Avoid it and live healthy and long!

Make a valiant attempt to discontinue the use of these devitalized foodless foods, toxic oils, and their products. Detox your liver with green vegetables, lemons, and these herbs: yucca, dandelion, milk thistle, barberry, Oregon grape root, and bilberry. These herbs and foods help to detox the fats and toxic chemical oils out of the liver and gallbladder, thus improving your vision. Your eyes will thank you for it. And you will have more energy than ever before!

Bad Effects of Rapeseed/Canola Oil and Soy Oil on Liver, Blood, Eyes, and Health

By John Thomas, author of Young Again!

The name *canola* is a coined word. Canola oil comes from the rapeseed, which is part of the mustard family of plants. Rape is the *most* toxic of all food oil plants. It is not listed in anything but the most recent reference sources. It is a word that appeared out of nowhere. Canola oil is a semi-drying oil that is used as a lubricant, in fuel, soap, rubber products, and magazine covers. Canola forms latexlike substances that cause agglutination of the red blood corpuscles, as does soy only MUCH more pronounced.

Loss of vision is a known characteristic side effect of rape (canola) oil. Rape antagonizes the central and peripheral nervous systems—like soy oil, only worse. Rape (canola) oil causes pulmo-

nary emphysema, respiratory distress, anemia, constipation, irritability, and blindness in the bodies of animals—and humans.

Rapeseed oil was in widespread use in animal feeds in England
and Europe between 1986 and 1991, when it was thrown out. Do
you remember reading about the cows, pigs, and sheep that went
blind, lost their minds, and attacked people? They had to be shot! . . .
The "experts" blamed the erratic behavior on a viral disease called
"scrapie." However, when rapeseed oil was removed from animal
feed, "scrapie" disappeared. Now we are growing rapeseed and
using rapeseed (canola) oil in the USA! Canola oil is now our problem. It is widely used in thousands of processed foods in the USA—
with the blessings of government watchdog agencies, of course!

Officially, canola oil is known as LEAR oil. The acronym stands for
"low erucic acid rape." The experts tell us it is "safe" to use. Through
genetic engineering, that is, irradiation, it is no longer rape, but instead
"canola"! The experts talk about canola's "qualities"—like its unsatu-
rated structure, omega 3, 6, and 12, its wonderful digestibility, and its
fatty acid makeup. They turn us against naturally saturated oils and
fats. . . . The term *canola* provided the perfect cover for commercial
interests who wanted to make billions in the USA. The name "canola"
is still in use, but it is no longer needed . . . look at the peanut butter
ingredient labels. The peanut oil has been removed and replaced with
rapeseed oil. Rapeseed oil is used to produce the chemical warfare
agent "mustard gas," used in all wars, including the recent Gulf War.

Canola oil contains large amounts of "iso-thio-cyanates," which are
cyanide compounds. Cyanide *inhibits* mitochondrial production of ade-
nosine triphosphate (ATP). ATP powers the body and keeps us healthy
and young. Notice the tremendous increase in disorders like systemic
lupus, multiple sclerosis, cerebral palsy, myelinoma, pulmonary hyper-
tension, and neuropathy in recent years. Soy and canola oils are players
in the development of these disease conditions. Canola oil is rich in
glycosides, which cause serious problems in the human body by blocking enzyme function and depriving us of our life force (chi, prana).

Soy and canola oil glycosides depress the immune system. They cause the white blood cell defense system—the T cells—to go into a stupor and fall asleep on the job. These oils alter the bio-electric "terrain" and promote disease. The alcohols and glycosides in canola and soy oils shut down our protective grid—the immune system.

In the movie *Lorenzo's Oil,* the dying boy had a chronically low total body pH. It was so low that his body fluids were dissolving the myelin sheath that protects the nerve fibers . . . causing his nervous system to disintegrate. The boy was given Lorenzo's oil to boost energy output and act as a detoxifier of metabolic poisons. The oil shocked his body into a less acid condition. Lorenzo's oil is *olive oil!* When given in large quantities, olive oil shocks the body and causes it to adjust its pH. It will also safely purge the body of gall and liver stones, thus avoiding the need for gallbladder surgery (yucca extract and PACs [proanthocyanidins] must precede the "flush"). On a TV talk show, an "expert" claimed that Lorenzo's oil was rapeseed oil. THIS WAS A LIE! Give rapeseed oil to a sick person and you will seal their doom. Here is another example of "disinformation" in the public domain. These falsehoods should cause every thinking person to question the molding of public opinion by powerful commercial interests behind the scenes . . . the astronomical increase in the use of processed foods that contain canola oil, soy oil, and chemical additives confuses the body and weakens the immune system.

The "health care" industry is an oxymoron. It protects its own economic interests. If you want peak health and longevity you *must* take control of your life, and be responsible for your own health. There is no other way!

Important Health Note on Oils—Caution! Read labels and watch for soy, canola, and cottonseed oil in thousands of food products! These toxic oils do not belong in the human blood system. They get sticky inside the body, cause clotting, blocked arteries, and untold damage to our health. Peanut oil is better on the skin than inside the body. Cottonseed oil is known to lower testosterone and sperm count in males! Read labels. Be informed. Take charge of your own health and healing!

Health Key Number 6: Use Healthy Oils Moderately for Good Vision and Health

Some vegetable oils are better than others for health and longevity. These include olive, sesame, sunflower, and flax oils. Olive is the Rolls Royce of oils! It comes from a fruit—the olive. Coconut oil is a medium chain fatty acid and excellent for your health, in spite of the dairy industry's campaign to give it a bad name. These oils are more stable and do not break down as fast as the dangerous oils discussed above. Vegans can use these healthful vegetable oils. Ghee (clarified butter) is excellent for cooking or on food. Keep all oils refrigerated after opening, except coconut oil—it can stay out indefinitely and not go bad! Other oils maintain their freshness in the fridge.

Do not consume excessive oils, even the good ones. A tablespoon or two in cooking or on salads is enough to lubricate your glands, hormones, and joints. Remember: you are not a car—you do not need five quarts of oil to run smoothly!

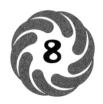

Complete Analysis of Nutritional Body Types and Protocol for Optimum Health and Perfect Eyesight

If we eat wrongly, no doctor can cure us. If we eat rightly, no doctor is needed.

VICTOR ROCINE

AYURVEDIC NUTRITIONAL BODY TYPING PROGRAM

In addition to avoiding unhealthy foods, it is important to consume the proper foods, herbs, vitamins, and supplements for your individual body type. The ayurvedic health system from India offers good guidance for high-level health and energy, and crystal clear vision. Ayurveda, or "life wisdom," addresses the three constitutional body types, or governing qualities within the body.

124

It is vitally important to know your individual body type, so that you will know what foods, herbs, and health protocol you require. It is a prerequisite to improving health and longevity and attaining perfect eyesight. Do not take this subject lightly. It can make the difference between excellent health and energy, or weakness, fatigue, and constant illness.

The three main body types are: *vata* (air-ectomorph-mental), *pitta* (fire-mesomorph-motive), and *kapha* (water-endomorph-vital).

The vata body type operates through the nervous system, colon, bones, and movement. Vata types are prone to dry, itchy eyes.

The pitta body type operates through the small intestines, digestion, and enzymatic and metabolic functions. Pitta types are prone to hot, inflamed, or red eyes.

The kapha body type operates through the respiratory system, lungs, body structure, and nutritive hormones. Kapha types are prone to watery, crusty, or expanded eyes.

A person can also be a combination of these main body types, exhibiting symptoms and characteristics of two body types, that is: kapha/pitta, pitta/vata, vata/pitta, or vata/kapha. In rare circumstances a person can be a combination of all three body types.

COMPLETE ANALYSIS AND PROTOCOL FOR THE KAPHA (WATER) BODY TYPE
(Watery, Crusty, Expanded Eyes)

You are a kapha (water) body type if you have excess mucus and crust in your eyes, especially in the morning; if your eyes tear, drip, and drain; if you discharge a lot of mucus from the nose and mouth, especially during cold weather; if you have colds and flu often; if you have chest and head congestion often. Water types usually have expanded watery kidneys and liver, which causes myopia or nearsightedness. You will also manifest the following characteristics and symptoms.

Characteristics of a Kapha (Water) Body Type

Large chest or breasts; large bones; overweight, strong physique; smooth, cold, thick skin; ease in gaining weight and difficulty in losing weight; thick, wavy hair; large forehead; thick eyebrows and eyelashes; large, wide nose; moist, oily lips; white, even teeth; pink, oily gums; wide, thick shoulders; thick, strong arms; big, moist, calm hands; large calves, feet, and joints; hard, thick, smooth, pale nails; milky, whitish urine; firm, mucus-filled feces once a day; medium-cool sweat and moderate body odor; moderate to low appetite—able to fast easily without hunger; round, deep, low voice; long-term memory; calm, sentimental emotions; conservative faith; slow, relaxed body movements; heavy, deep sleep; seldom dreams or have watery, romantic dreams; great endurance; enduring sexual energy; liking for children; strong immune system—quick to heal; prone to colds, flu, edema, asthma, bronchitis, pneumonia, and so on; slow digestion; pulse: 60–70 (slow, even, steady, swan-like beat); large, round, watery, calm eyes; cold, damp, bloated, heavy stomach; low hunger; dull, heavy pain; low grade fever; swollen, watery, expanded throat; sleepy after eating; anal itch; excess urine, but less frequent.

Healthy kapha (water) types may only experience these symptoms occasionally or not at all. The healthier you are, the less watery symptoms you will experience. Follow the protocol suggestions of reducing water, and you will be delighted with the results.

Kapha (Water) Body Types Need Less Water, Not More!

Just drink when you are thirsty. Overdrinking of water, juice, or other liquids waterlogs the body and causes bloating, weight gain, and fatigue. Excess water in the body manifests in water body types as watery, crusty eyes, edema, and obesity. Drink less water during cold, damp weather. High humidity causes water retention in cells, tissues, and eyes.

The kidneys, bladder, and adrenals are weakened by excess liquid intake. This can cause incontinence (weak bladder), poor eyesight, waterlogging of the brain, mental confusion, reduction of stomach acids, which results in stomach bloating, water-weight-gain, yin or expanded kidneys, and cold hands and feet. The benefit of drinking excess water to "flush-out" the body is a fallacy! Precious adrenal (energy hormones) are urinated out when the body is loaded with water. The body is a self-regulating, self-healing natural organism. You need rest, proper sleep, exercise, natural foods, and pure oxygen to heal and keep your body healthy. Too much water only weakens the system and causes weak internal organs and illness. Don't fall for the "half-a-gallon-a-day-water-drinking-delusion." Drink when thirsty and stop. There are no health benefits to be gained by trying to "force-flush" the kidneys and lymph system.

The kidneys, bladder, and lymph require the proper balance of food, water, exercise, and rest. Overdoing any one of these natural body requirements is the cause of much illness and disease. Moderation and balance in diet and habits is the key to good health and improved vision.

Potato Juice Eye Bath for Watery Eyes

Eyes that water easily and form crusts overnight can benefit tremendously from a daily three-minute Potato Juice Bath. Grate a raw potato and squeeze the juice out through a cheesecloth or strainer. Squeeze enough juice to fill an eyecup, about two to three teaspoons. Place the eyecup, filled with potato juice, over each eye and hold it there for three minutes. Tilt head back or lie down on your back. Try to keep your eye open and the cup held firmly around the eye.

Avoid These Foods if You Have Watery Eyes

If you have many of the above characteristics, you are a water body type and prone to watery eyes. Kapha (water) body types must avoid the following watery, moist foods: fruit, juices, milk, yogurt, soy oil, canola oil, safflower oil, peppermint, wintergreen, spearmint, licorice, zucchini, banana, beef, salt (a half ounce of salt holds four pounds of water in the body for weeks), sweets, melons, cucumber, tofu, coconut, grapes, dates, figs, tomatoes.

Avoid any foods, liquids, supplements, or condiments that tend to create water or mucus in your eyes and body. If you are living in a hot dry climate, some of these raw watery foods will be acceptable. But limit them in cold, damp wintry weather.

Foods that Reduce Water and Mucus for the Kapha (Water) Body Type

Kapha (water) types need foods that reduce water, dry up mucus, and balance and harmonize the system. For best results, foods must be boiled, baked, broiled, steamed, or sautéed. Such foods will give your body the necessary warmth and dryness to reduce weight and fat. The foods listed below are loaded with vitamins and minerals, and will fire up your metabolism, control your weight, improve your digestion, and strengthen your eyesight.

Ninety percent of your food should be low-calorie grains, steamed green vegetables, and light vegetable broth soups. Regularly eat plenty of the following drying foods to reduce fat, mucus, and water in your body cells, tissues, and brain, which will allow your eyes to function at their best: baked potatoes; yams; squash; popcorn; toasted bread; low-fat and low-salt corn, potato, or rice chips; baked casseroles. In the winter consume more cooked vegetables, lean protein or vegetarian protein, whole grains, pastas, soups, root vegetables, and spices; in the summer eat a little more raw salads and fruit.

These fruits are good for kapha types: cherries and berries (raspberries, blueberries, blackberries). You can cook or stew these fruits. Dried fruit is better than fresh fruit. Grapes are also good for strengthening and cleansing the liver. Eat them during summer and fall seasons, but not during winter. Especially avoid: cucumbers, strawberries, watermelons, and all other melons. Or you can avoid fruit altogether, especially in the winter. Fruit is high in water, which is the main cause of eye mucus and tissue waterlogging.

Many children develop vision problems as a result of excess mucus in the body. To remedy this condition, use one clove of garlic every day, or take one or two Kyolic garlic capsules, especially during late winter and early spring—February through May—a damp, wet, and mucus-causing season for water body types.

Eat "just enough" spices to reduce mucus and water. Too many spices in the diet can cause eye inflammation or red eyes in any body type.

COMPLETE DIETARY REQUIREMENTS FOR THE KAPHA (WATER) BODY TYPE
Foods, Herbs, Vitamins, Minerals, and Supplements

Vegetables: Artichoke, arrowroot, asparagus, beets, beet greens, bitter melon, broccoli, brussels sprouts, burdock, cabbage, carrots, celery, cauliflower, Chinese cabbage, bok choy, cilantro, corn, collard greens, dandelion greens, eggplant, endive, fennel, anise, potatoes, green beans, green peppers, horseradish, kale, kohlrabi, leeks, lotus root, mushrooms, mustard greens, onions, okra, parsley, pumpkin, parsnips, peas, red pepper, scallions, turnips, spinach, sprouts, swiss chard, baked squash and sweet potato (yams), cooked tomatoes, watercress, seaweed.

Fruit: Apples, apricots, blueberries, cherries, currants, grapefruit, kiwi, papaya, peaches, pineapple, pomegranate, cranberries, prunes, raspberries, blackberries, huckleberries, lemons, limes.

Grains: Corn, millet, oats, rice, rye, wheat, sago, spelt, kamut, amaranth, muesli, couscous, quinoa, oat bran, tapioca, whole-grain pasta, rice cakes, dry cereals, basmati rice, wild rice, polenta.

Legumes: These are perfect protein foods for kapha types: black-eyed peas, lentils, yellow or green split peas, dried green peas, chickpeas, kidney beans, lima beans, navy beans, pinto beans. (Eat beans for protein if you are a vegetarian.) The Naturade Company sells an excellent soy-free Vegetarian Protein Powder, which you can add to your soups, dressings, and sauces.

Dairy: Low-fat and nonfat cottage cheese or cheese, ghee, goat milk, nonfat yogurt. Use dairy infrequently or during hot weather or in dry hot climate or in autumn (dry hot season).

Animal Protein: Chicken, turkey, eggs, freshwater fish. Use these foods moderately.

Seeds: Sunflower, sesame, poppy, pumpkin, chia, flax.

Nuts: Almonds, cashews, pecans, walnuts, pistachios, filberts, hazelnuts. (Only eat nuts in small quantities, and only if they are dry roasted or soaked in water overnight.)

Oils: Flax, sesame, olive, sunflower, ghee.

Sweeteners: Raw honey, molasses, rice syrup.

Condiments and Spices: Allspice, anise, apple cider vinegar, asafetida, basil, bay leaf, black pepper, caraway, cayenne, chili peppers, chives, cinnamon, cloves, cress, cumin, dill, fennel, garlic, ginger (dry powder), mace, marjoram, mustard, neem leaves, nutmeg, oregano, parsley, pumpkin pie spice, rosemary, sage, savory, thyme, tarragon, turmeric.

Beverages: Dry wines, aloe vera gel, apple cider, apple juice, apricot juice, berry juice, black tea (spiced), cherry juice, cranberry juice, grain coffee, Dacopa, mango juice, vegetable juice, peach juice, pomegranate juice, prune juice, rice milk, almond milk. (Consume juices sparingly and mostly during hot weather.)

Herbal Teas: Alfalfa, blackberry, borage, burdock, catnip, chamomile, chicory, clove, chrysanthemum, cinnamon, corn silk, dandelion, eyebright tea (for all eye conditions), bilberry (for nearsightedness and night vision), elder flower, eucalyptus, fennel, fenugreek, juniper berry, oat straw, nettle, orange peel, raspberry, red clover, saffron, sage, sassafras, yerba maté, Good Earth Traditionals—Cinnamon Spice and Vanilla Spice.

Food Supplements: Bee pollen, honey, royal jelly, spirulina, alfalfa seed tablets, green kamut.

Vitamins: A, B, B$_{12}$, C, D, E, F.

Minerals: Sulfur, carbon, hydrogen, chlorine, iron, magnesium, chromium, selenium.

Protein: 10–20 percent daily intake.

Carbohydrates: 70–80 percent daily intake: grains, vegetables.

Fats: 10–15 percent daily intake.

Special Therapies to Balance Kapha (Water) Body Type

- Diet emphasizing the three water-reducing tastes: pungent, bitter, astringent.
- Periodic fasting from food and too much liquid.
- Herbal elixirs.
- Hot dry heat. Dry saunas—up to forty-five minutes, three to four times a week—are excellent to dry up water and mucus in your body. Or live in a dry climate, like that of Arizona.
- Emetic therapy to clear mucus out of the stomach.
- Dry, deep massage with lotions made up of hot herbs like ginger, mustard oil, onion, and asafetida.
- Breathing exercises that create heat in the body, such as deep yogic breathing through your right nostril.
- Chi Kung moving and breathing exercises.
- Plenty of vigorous exercise, forty-five to sixty minutes daily, such as: walking, running, biking, low-impact weight-bearing aerobic activity, high-repetition and low-weight resistance barbells, dumbbells, or machines, stair climbers, treadmills, mountain climbing, stair climbing, step-ups.
- Reduced sleep time. Avoid oversleeping—it causes weight gain.

COMPLETE ANALYSIS AND PROTOCOL FOR THE VATA (AIR) BODY TYPE
(Dry, Twitching, Itchy, and Contracted Eyes)

You are a vata (air) body type if you suffer from problems manifested by dryness and twitching eyes, dry, dull, flaky skin, thin or underweight body, dry hair, dry cough, and constant digestive problems. You will also manifest the following characteristics and symptoms.

Characteristics of a Vata (Air) Body Type

Small, narrow shoulders and sunken chest; thin, dry, rough, jittery, nervous hands; dry feet; cracking joints; dry, brittle, thin, rough, discolored nails with deep ridges; dry, hard, scant bowel movements; gas, painful constipation; inconsistent, irregular, or no appetite for days; low, frail, rasping voice; fast, shifting, rambling, weak voice; changeable, fast, uncertain, indecisive, and easily excitable; poor memory; hyperactive, accident-prone; ungrounded gait; irregular eating and sleeping patterns; insomnia; weak muscles; tire easily; low immune response; constant fatigue; bone aches, arthritis; spinal abnormalities; schizophrenia (paranoia); paralysis; Parkinson's disease; rheumatism; ear ringing; fissures of anus, nipple; tics, tremors, twitches; heart palpitations; congenital giantism or dwarfism; bowlegged or knock-kneed; impatience, restlessness; vacillation and indecisiveness; poor self-image; intolerance to cold weather and cold drinks; undue dependence on others; enthusiasm followed by depression; weak digestion; pulse: 80 or over (narrow and slithery); dry mouth, throat; fearful, apathetic, loner.

Avoid These Foods if You Have Dry Eyes

If you have many of the above characteristics, you are an air body type and prone to dry eyes. Avoid any foods or condiments that tend to create dryness in your system. This is especially true if you are a pitta/vata dual body type, in which case you may exhibit pitta heat or fire symptoms with vata dryness and thinness. Dry vata (air) body types must avoid the following dry foods: dry toast, breads (unless steamed soft), crackers, chips, corn chips, dried fruits, baked foods, hot condiments such as dry ginger powder, curry, hot peppers, cayenne pepper.

If, however, you exhibit signs of coldness and dampness combined with a vata body type, you must avoid cold, damp food, juices, raw food, and fruit in cold weather. You should eat more dry and warming foods and some spices for balance.

Warming, Moisturizing, Grounding Foods to Balance the Vata (Air) Body Type

Ninety percent of your food should be cooked (boiled, steamed, sautéed, broiled) to give your body the necessary warming moisture, vitamins, and minerals, which in turn will boost your hormones, digestion, strength, and eyesight. Eat thick soups and natural puddings such as rice pudding, squash or yam puddings, and so on. Non-vegetarian vata types can get protein from organically raised chicken, turkey, or salmon, or goat milk and goat cheese. Vegan or vegetarian vata types can eat hemp protein, brown rice protein powder, soaked seeds and nuts, imported nutritional yeast, or yellow flaked nutritional yeast, Vegetarian Protein Powder from Naturade, fava beans, lima beans, garbanzo beans, and chickpea sauce. These are warming, moisturizing, and nurturing to build and nourish your hormones, cells, tissues, brain, and eyes. Eat plenty of these foods regularly.

Vata (air) body types need to eat more sour, sweet, and moisturizing foods during October, November, December, and January—when the weather has a drying effect on the body and eyes. Eat more soups, steamed and boiled vegetables, grains, and beans in cold weather. In autumn eat a little more oils and sour foods such as: yogurt, apple cider vinegar, lemons, thick cabbage soups, beets, and goat milk to counteract the dryness of the season. Reduce oils and fats in hot summer months. Eat more protein in winter and less in summer.

Eat a bit more raw fruits and vegetables in hot summer weather. Grapes are excellent for strengthening and cleansing the liver. They help to improve eyesight. Eat them mainly during the summer and fall months. They are too cooling to eat during winter in the north. If you are cold, with gas, bloating, and indigestion, stay away from fruit altogether in cold weather. Raw fruits and vegetables, eaten in cold weather, make the stomach cold; this creates a stomach pH over 7.5, much too alkaline and cold to generate heat, digestive juices, and overall grounding and warmth.

The stomach is like a pot; it must maintain a 100-degree temperature to rot, process, and digest food properly. Without stomach heat, vata types suffer from indigestion, gas, bloating, weight loss, and fatigue. A 100 percent raw food diet is not good for thin vata types— it is too light, airy, and cold to maintain their weight and health. A person of the vata type needs to warm their stomach or central energy with cooked grains, thick soups, and root vegetables to maintain balance.

Important Note: Too many dried foods will cause dry eyes. Choose your foods wisely and "see" your vision improve daily.

COMPLETE DIETARY REQUIREMENTS FOR THE VATA (AIR) BODY TYPE
Foods, Herbs, Vitamins, Minerals, and Supplements

Vegetables: Beets, carrots, parsnips, peas, seaweed, sweet potatoes (yams), pumpkin, onions, green beans, squash (winter), asparagus, occasional greens.

Fruits: Apricots, blueberries, cherries, coconut, dates, figs, kiwi, lemons, limes, oranges, currants, pineapple, prunes, mangoes, peaches, apples, and applesauce. Eat fruit mainly in warm summer weather, otherwise you may overcleanse, lose weight, thin your blood, and get cold hands and feet in the winter.

Grains: Oats, wheat, rice, spelt, and amaranth.

Legumes: Make soups from these foods: lentils, lima beans, yellow and green split peas, chickpeas, black-eyed peas, green peas, navy beans, and kidney beans.

Seeds: Pumpkin, sesame (and tahini), sunflower, flax.

Nuts: Almonds, cashews, pecans, walnuts—all soaked overnight or cooked in food.

Dairy: Goat milk yogurt, butter (ghee), raw goat milk, goat milk cheese.

Animal and Vegetarian Protein: Amish chicken, fish, lamb (occasional and only 5 percent of diet). Vegetarians use goat milk, organic goat cheese, and goat milk yogurt; soy-free Vegetarian Protein Powder by Naturade, imported nutritional yeast grown on beet molasses by Kal.

Oils: Olive, sesame, sunflower, flax.

Sweeteners: Maple syrup, rice syrup, fruit juice (in warm weather only).

Condiments and Spices: Almond extract, anise, basil, cardamom, cinnamon, coriander, cumin, dill, fennel, marjoram, parsley, poppy seeds, rosemary, savory, tarragon; Bragg's Liquid Aminos, No Salt Spike, Dr. Bronner's Mineral Seasoning.

Beverages: Almond milk, rice milk, Dacopa or grain "coffee," lemonade, mango juice, peach juice.

Herbal Teas: Licorice, orange peel, saffron, sarsaparilla, chamomile, Good Earth Tea (Original), Yogi Teas.

Food Supplements: Aloe vera juice internally and externally (a few drops in the eyes morning and night).

Minerals: Calcium, copper, iron, zinc, magnesium.

Protein: 25–30 percent daily intake.

Carbohydrates: 50 percent daily intake: grains, vegetables, pasta.

Fats: 15–20 percent daily intake.

Special Therapies to Increase Moisture and Warmth in Vata (Air) Body Types

- Diet emphasizing the three tastes that increase moisture and warmth in the body: sweet, sour, salty.
- Small, frequent meals—never overeat or overstuff stomach.
- More oil in diet. Sesame oil on skin.
- Herbal elixirs: Dracsha, Restora, Chavranprash, and Dashmula are all good for vata conditions, that is, related to the nerves, kidneys, and eyesight. They impart strength, energy, endurance, and rejuvenation.
- Herbal teas that warm and strengthen the body: rosemary, ginseng, ashwangandha, licorice, marshmallow, ginger, cinnamon, Good Earth Teas—Cinnamon Spice and Vanilla Spice.
- Warm, moist steam baths or water.
- Oil enema.
- Gentle oil massage.
- Massage feet with mustard oil during fall and winter to improve eyesight and warm the body; massage at night before bed to sleep soundly.
- Soft, relaxing music.
- Healing, warming, and strengthening colors: red, yellow, orange, green, magenta, scarlet.
- Knee, ankle, wrist wraps, or lifting belt for injured or prolapsed limb or organs.
- Yoga alternate-nostril breathing, performed slowly and smoothly.

- Exercise using soft, gentle movements such as yoga stretching, Tai Chi, Chi Kung breathing, walking outdoors in the forest, lake, or countryside, light weightlifting—ten to twenty minutes, three times a week.
- Calm meditation that soothes the nervous system.

COMPLETE ANALYSIS AND PROTOCOL FOR THE PITTA (FIRE) BODY TYPE
(Hot, Stinging, Red Inflamed Eyes, or Conjunctivitis)

Whether you are a watery-eyed water body type or a dried-eyed air body type, you can still suffer from inflamed, red eyes if you eat too many sweets, fats, and hot spicy foods. However, the pitta (fire) body type is more prone to hot, red, inflamed eyes. You will also manifest the following characteristics and symptoms.

Characteristics of a Pitta (Fire) Body Type

Muscular toned body; red stinging eyes; flushed or red face; acne, freckles, and moles; early graying and balding; piercing eyes with red lines; soft, pink, bleeding gums; yellow/red, profuse, or burning urine with strong odor; diarrhea, loose stools; excess, hardy, sharp appetite, but still thin; sharp, piercing voice; critical, forceful bearing, stubborn; short, clear memory; angry, jealous, edgy emotions; fiery leader; colorful dreams; motivated, driven; strong passions, obsessions; dislikes heat, tends to infections, inflammations, tumors, rashes, fevers, skin disorders; yellow-coated tongue; reacts strongly to medicine; pulse: 70–80 (strong, jumpy); hot, strong stomach energy, fast digestion; burning and heat in chest and head after eating hot, spicy, pungent foods; burning, inflamed throat; emotions can go from extreme joy and laughter to extreme despair and depression.

Avoid These Foods if You Have Inflamed, Red, Stinging Eyes

If you have many of the above characteristics, you are a fire body type and prone to red stinging eyes. Hot pitta (fire) body types must avoid the following dry foods: garlic, hot peppers, raw onions, cayenne pepper, curry, egg yolk, chips of all kinds, nuts (unless soaked overnight and small amount), millet, corn, rye, chicken and turkey, lentils, goat milk, wheat, black pepper, cloves, chives, ginger, nutmeg, corn oil, soy oil, canola oil, safflower oil, almond oil, bee pollen, royal jelly.

Foods to Cool and Balance the Pitta (Fire) Body Type

Forty to 60 percent of your food should be raw, that is, fruits and vegetables with cooling minerals, vitamins, enzymes, fiber, and water to keep your hormones, cells, tissues, brain, and eyes cool and functioning at their best.

Sour and sweet foods are beneficial moistening foods. If the weather is hot and dry, eat more cooling fruits and vegetables and drink cooling fresh juice drinks or pure water. June, July, August, and September are the months of the fiery hot season for most of the country. In the southwest United States dry hot weather prevails most of the time, and you will need to consume more cooling, raw, and moistening foods and liquids if you live there. Eat the foods grown in your own area and climate, and you can't go too far wrong.

Eat a little more soups, steamed and boiled vegetables, grains, and beans in cold weather. Eat oils or dairy more in autumn to counteract the dryness of the season. Consume less oils and fats in hot summer months. Eat more raw fruits and vegetables in hot summer weather. Grapes are an excellent food for the liver and should be eaten mainly during the summer and fall months. They are too cooling to eat during northern winter months. Eat a little more protein in winter and less in summer.

COMPLETE DIETARY REQUIREMENTS FOR THE PITTA (FIRE) BODY TYPE
Foods, Herbs, Vitamins, Minerals, and Supplements

Vegetables: Arrowroot, artichoke, asparagus, beets, beet greens, bitter melon, broccoli, brussels sprouts, cabbage, carrots, cauliflower, celery, okra, cilantro, cucumber, dandelion greens, fennel, anise, green beans, kale, Swiss chard, collard greens, lettuce—bib, Boston, romaine, and other leaf lettuces (avoid head lettuce as it has very little nutritional value), olives, mushrooms, Chinese cabbage, bok choy, endive, radish, parsley, peas, rutabaga, tomatoes, turnips, watercress, squash, sweet potato.

Fruits: Avocados, blackberries, cantaloupe, sweet apples, applesauce, coconut, soaked currants, grapes, melons, papaya, peaches, pears, persimmons, pomegranates, soaked raisins, rhubarb, raspberries, strawberries, soaked dates, watermelon, sweet cherries, soaked figs, limes, mangoes, sweet oranges, sweet pineapple, sweet plums, soaked prunes.

Grains: Barley, buckwheat, oats, rice, spelt, oat bran, sago, tapioca, amaranth, kamut.

Legumes: Adzuki beans, black beans, black-eyed peas, green peas, lima beans, mung beans and sprouts, navy beans, chickpeas, kidney beans, pinto beans.

Dairy: Soft cheese, butter, ghee, cottage cheese, yogurt, skim milk.

Animal Protein: Egg whites, shrimp, fish, tuna, halibut, white fish, salmon. These foods all have neutral to cooling energy. Keep animal foods 5–10 percent of diet.

Seeds: Pumpkin, sunflower, sesame.

Oils: Sesame, olive, flax, sunflower.

Sweeteners: Barley malt, fruit juice, rice syrup.

Condiments and Spices: Basil, coriander, cress, dill, marjoram, miso, parsley, peppermint, gray moist sea salt, savory, seaweed (hijiki, kombu), spearmint, tarragon, thyme, wintergreen.

Beverages: Almond milk, aloe vera juice, apple juice, apricot juice, blueberry juice, blackberry juice, black tea, carob drink, cherry juice, grain coffee, grape juice, mango juice, vegetable juice, peach juice, pear juice, pomegranate juice, cranberry juice, prune juice, rice milk, Dacopa.

Herbal teas: Alfalfa, barley, burdock, chamomile, chrysanthemum and honeysuckle (both are used internally and externally for inflamed eyes), jasmine, hibiscus, rehmania (raw), lavender, lemon balm, licorice, oat straw, peppermint, red clover.

Food Supplements: Spirulina, blue green algae, green kamut, green chlorella, alfalfa tablets. Chavranprash with saffron is a good ayurvedic tonic paste for pitta conditions.

Vitamins: A, B, B$_{12}$, C, K, U, bioflavonoids.

Minerals: Copper, iron, potassium, magnesium.

Protein: 20 percent daily intake.

Carbohydrates: 60–70 percent daily intake.

Fats: 15–20 percent daily intake.

Important Note for Pitta (Fire) Types: Too many hot spicy foods can cause red inflamed eyes and hot blood. Make wise choices of foods for your fire body type, and you will "see" your vision improve quickly.

Special Therapies to Reduce Heat and Inflammation in Pitta (Fire) Body Types

- Diet emphasizing the four tastes to reduce heat and inflammation in the body: sweet, bitter, astringent, salty.
- Purgation therapy. Use aloe vera, dandelion, senna, yellow dock, cascara sagrada.

- Avoid excess heat. Apply herbal sprays, cool lotions, pastes, and oils made from sandalwood, lavender, rose petals, aloe vera, and so on.
- Ghee (clarified butter) internally and applied externally on body.
- Healing, cooling, and calming colors: blue, purple, turquoise, magenta.
- Practice slow breathing techniques such as yoga and Chi Kung to cool and calm the body.
- Perform yoga bending movements that tone the small intestines.
- Exercise during the cool part of the day. Get lots of outdoor activity and oxygen. Swimming, walking, running, sports, mountain climbing, biking. Light weightlifting—do not strain or overtrain while lifting weights. Non-impact aerobic exercises are also beneficial. Remember not to get too over-heated when exercising, as it could raise blood pressure and heart rate.
- Calming and quiet meditation by lakes, oceans, trees, and mountains, to bring peace and calmness to mind and body.

The Chinese five-element health system overlaps with the ayurvedic system. It addresses the five pairs of internal organs, their relationship to each other, the correct five food tastes for each organ, and the condition of each organ system—is it warm, hot, neutral, cold, or cool? We will cover both systems and their relationships thoroughly in a future book.

We recommend that you study both kinds of body typing principles in other books on ayurveda and Chinese medicine. When you study and practice this way of eating and living, you will develop intuition and insight. You'll know automatically what foods you require at any given time. You'll know also when to eat, when to fast or cleanse, how much to exercise, rest, and sleep.

To begin, follow the suggestions given above as best you can. If you fall off the program for a day or a week, get right back on it. After eating the correct foods for your individual body type, you will feel a new surge of power and focus. Your body and mind will become balanced and grounded. Above all, your health and energy will increase by leaps and bounds. And so will your vision.

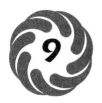

Do You Really Want Perfect Eyesight?

Some people think about improving their eyesight, but no one ever improved their vision just by thinking. Thinking and reading about eyesight improvement is merely the first step on the road to perfect eyesight. Many like to talk about improving their vision, but you can talk until you're "blue in the face," with zero results. Others haphazardly practice the exercises. Of course, they receive little or no results.

Vision improvement comes only from regular, consistent practice, correctly performed. You can achieve this for yourself by following the instructions and suggestions given in this book, outlined below.

NATURAL WAYS TO PERFECT EYESIGHT OUTLINE

In the 1930s Dr. Alexis Carroll from the Rockefeller Medical Institute wrote a classic book entitled *Man the Unknown*. Dr. Carroll kept a chicken heart alive for twenty years in a petri dish by following a procedure that included: 1) proper nutrition; 2) proper elimination; and 3) good circulation or exercise.

We can improve our own vision and health by following the same example as Dr. Carroll in this manner.

1. Nourish the eyes with nutrient-dense organic foods, supplements, and herbs.
2. Clear toxins from the eyes, liver, stomach, and colon by eating properly, following good health habits, and undergoing periodic cleansing diets or elimination fasts.
3. Strengthen the eye muscles with specific eye improvement exercises.

1. Feed the Eyes

- Eat wholesome nutritious foods for your body type, following the suggestions given in chapter 8.
- Use natural, whole-food vitamins, minerals, and herbs (see chapter 7).
- "Feed" your eyes by Sunning them (see chapter 2).
- Eat only when hungry; don't overeat.
- Drink only when thirsty.

2. Methods of Cleansing the Eyes of Toxins

- Stop eating junk foods, transfats, margarine, aspartame, sucralose, sugar, white flour, white rice, commercial dairy, and fast food.
- Use an eyecup to bathe your eyes with lemon juice (or apple cider vinegar, or cayenne) in water (see chapter 3).
- Do Yoga Nasal Massage with finger and sesame oil or one drop of eucalyptus or lavender oil (see chapter 3).
- Cleanse the liver with an elimination detox diet or "fasting," on fruits and vegetables, vegetable juices, dandelion root, eyebright, lutein, barberry, bilberry, milk thistle, bupleurum, chrysanthemum, and other herbal teas.

- Use the healing sound sh-h-h-h-h-h-h to purify your liver and eyes; visualize the color green and kindness while inhaling, and exhale anger and unkindness (see chapter 5).
- Use Do-In Self-Massage to clear blockages (see chapter 6).
- Exercise overall body three to four times per week; walk outdoors one to two miles per day.

3. Strengthen the Eye Muscles with Eye Exercises

Because of our busy schedules—trying to make a living, raising children, or going to school—we have less time for eye exercises. But you will see results in improved vision if you use our special Short Eye Exercise Routine, which takes only about fifteen minutes, three times a week. Compare that to how much time you spend in front of the "brainwashing device" (your TV). Surely you can find forty-five minutes a week to maintain healthy eyes and prevent eye problems in the future. If you have more time, use the Medium Eye Exercise Routine, with two eye sessions a week, of at least forty minutes each. Set a regular time for your eye sessions and stick to it! Detailed instructions for the exercises and techniques in these routines are given in chapters 2, 3, 4, and 5.

EYE ROUTINES FOR THOSE WITH BUSY SCHEDULES

Short Eye Exercise Routine

Fifteen minutes, three times a week

- Egyptian Black Dot exercise: five minutes
- Tai Chi Rocker exercise: five minutes
- Eye Palming technique: five minutes
- Reaching for Heaven exercise: six times every morning

Medium Eye Exercise Routine

Forty minutes, two times a week

- Warm-up exercises such as neck rolls and eye massages: two to three minutes
- Egyptian Black Dot exercise: five minutes
- Stretch Your Vision exercise for myopia or Close Vision Strengthening exercises for presbyopia: fifteen minutes
- Tai Chi Rocker exercise: five minutes
- Tibetan Peripheral Vision technique: five minutes
- Eye Palming technique: five minutes
- Chi Kung exercises: five minutes

EXTENDED EYESIGHT TRAINING EXERCISE SCHEDULE

If your schedule allows, your eyesight will be benefited if you build up to a more extensive training program. Detailed instructions for the following exercises and techniques are given in chapters 2, 3, 4, and 5.

Extended Eye Exercise Routine

One hour plus, two or three times a week

- Warm-up exercises such as neck rolls and head, face, and eye massages: three minutes
- Eye Muscle exercises: five to ten minutes
- Tibetan Peripheral Vision technique: five minutes
- Distance Seeing exercises for nearsightedness or Close Seeing exercises for farsightedness: fifteen to thirty minutes
- Chi Kung exercises: fifteen minutes
- Eye Palming technique: five to ten minutes

EASY NO-ROUTINE NATURAL EYE EXERCISES

There are also many eye exercises that you can work into your spare moments throughout each day. They are not only helpful but also fun!

 ## Easy Distance Vision Strengthening Exercises

- Focus your vision on a bird in flight.
- Focus your vision on a moving ball or object at sporting events.
- Practice juggling a ball.
- Gaze at a moving car until it is out of sight.
- Track or edge distant objects, such as cars, trees, houses, letters, signs, and so on.
- Gaze as far as you can see into the horizon, or at the night stars.
- Gaze relaxedly at nature's bounty—trees, flowers, lakes, oceans, grass, and so on.
- Gaze at the night moon. Look at the red rising or setting sun.

Easy Exercises to Boost Close Vision

- Gaze at a tiny period for 20 seconds.
- Look up from your close work regularly (every five to ten minutes).
- Perform the Eye Palming technique often throughout the day.
- Close eyes often and relax your mind and thoughts.
- Trace close objects or letters 20 inches or less away from you.

Easy Peripheral Vision Strengthening Exercises

- When walking or traveling in your car, notice the surrounding objects moving toward you and past you.
- While looking straight ahead, observe objects to your left, right, up, and down. Do not move your eyes. See objects with your peripheral vision only.

 ## Easy Pupil Strengthening Exercises

- Go outside; cover your eyes for 2 seconds; next, uncover your eyes for 2 seconds. Keep your eyes open throughout this entire pupil exercise. Perform this exercise for 1 or 2 minutes.
- Sit next to a light switch; turn light on for 1 second, then turn light off for 3 or 4 seconds. Perform this exercise for 2 minutes.

DAILY EYE HEALTH PROGRAM

For excellent eye health, also practice the following daily:

1. Hold your reading material at least twenty inches from your eyes.
2. Sit and stand with a good posture.
3. Obtain sufficient rest and sleep.
4. Go outside daily in the fresh air and sunshine.
5. Go outside or take a slow walk after eating.
6. Perform the Head Lift technique.

Eye Exercises and Moderation: How Much Is Enough?

Eye exercises practiced in *moderation* improve vision faster than over-exercising or underexercising the eyes. Never perform the eye routine if your eyes are sore or aching from the previous eye routine. Let them rest a few days before performing another eye routine.

The eyes and body heal during rest periods. That's why we recommend one, two, or three days of rest between eye sessions, depending on how quickly your eyes respond after the routine. If you have the energy and vitality to perform eye exercises three times a week, by all means do so. One or two days a week is also good if you are pressed for time.

Do not exercise your eyes when you are sleepy, tired, fatigued, or when your eyes are red, itchy, watery, or inflamed. The greatest cause of poor eyesight is reading when tired, sleepy, and fatigued, especially at night before bedtime. The best time to perform your eye routine is when you are full of energy and rested in body and mind. You'll get the best results when you are refreshed, energetic, and looking forward to your next eye routine.

Deep undisturbed sleep allows the body to heal the eyes. If you are refreshed and "jump" out of bed after five or six hours of deep sleep, that is all your body needs. If you need eight hours to wake up refreshed, then make sure you get eight hours of solid, undisturbed sleep. Remember that fatigue, lethargy, mental confusion, low blood sugar, and depression are all precursor symptoms to chronic, degenerative disease, including debilitating eye problems.

Successful Eyesight Training Stories

Woman Does Eye Routine Only Once a Week and Improves Her Vision Dramatically!

Even with a once-a-week eye routine your vision can be improved substantially! Kaye Gowman of Royal Oak, Michigan, performs eye exercises only once a week with excellent results. She improved her eyesight from 20–400 (advanced myopia), to better than 20–20 in a few years on this limited eye routine. She really enjoys her eye routine because of the satisfaction of clear sight and the fact that she no longer needs burdensome eyeglasses or contacts. There is no excuse for not doing eye exercises, because even one eye routine a week can give you good results. Get started! What are you waiting for?

Lady Throws Glasses Away after Only One Eyesight Training Session

Stephanie Peterson of Ferndale, Michigan, was absolutely delighted after just one private eye training session with Robert Zuraw. Before she came to the eye-training session she wore contacts and glasses to correct her 20–100 vision. After an hour of performing specific eye exercises, she no longer required glasses to read or drive her car home. She was totally amazed at the results of just one session of natural perfect eyesight training. She actually "screamed for joy" as she got into her car.

PERFORM THE EYE ROUTINES WITH FUN, JOY, AND RELAXATION

This is an important point to burn into your memory; never forget it: the more relaxed we are, the better our vision becomes. Eye exercises performed mechanically, without focused attention, will not improve your vision. Perfect eyesight requires total relaxation of the body, mind, and eye muscles. Be in the moment and be aware of each movement. Relax the eye muscles, let go of mouth and facial muscles, hands, and shoulders. Feel these areas soft and relaxed—let go of hardness and tightness. Eyesight improves more quickly and easily with relaxation and focused attention.

Practice yoga with a good teacher and learn to feel what it's like to be totally relaxed, grounded, and centered. You can also relax with a shiatsu massage, Rolfing treatment, or any type of good deep massage technique.

Stress Affects Vision

When problems overwhelm us, we tend not to look clearly at objects or the world, as if we are blocking out life. As a result, we stop using our focusing muscles, and our vision weakens. A stressful situation that lasts for months or years is bound to weaken our vision drastically. However, it's only when we "stop looking" (stop using our eye-focusing muscles) that we lose our eyesight. When we practice the eye exercises and eye habits, the eyes continue to focus, regardless of how much stress we have. We can handle more stress without it harming our vision. Then, when our life gets back to a normal relaxed state, it becomes much easier to improve our vision.

EYE RELAXATION TIPS FOR BETTER VISION

Avoid Squinting

Learn to see without muscular effort. The eyes naturally squint in bright light, snow, or water reflection. Other than that, squinting to read or see an object will only weaken your eyesight. Avoid squinting by consciously relaxing your eyebrows. Soften your eyebrows and see without effort. Let outer objects come to your vision with ease. Avoid looking with a hard gaze. When your vision is perfect (40–10 or better), squinting will not occur, even in bright light or snow reflections.

Some people tense the muscles below the brow, just above the eyeball, at the inside of the nose bridge. Myopics develop this bad habit from too much close work. These muscles need to become soft and relaxed in order to see in the distance clearly. Here is an easy exercise to relax the eyebrows.

Arch the Eyebrows

Raise the eyebrows and consciously open the eyes wider, while maintaining a relaxed look. This allows you to see more comfortably and easily into the distance without squinting.

Too Much Close Work—Use Your Distant Vision

If you sit in front of a computer, read, or perform other close work, be sure to look up from your close work every five to ten minutes. Look out the window if possible. In addition, practice distant seeing while walking and driving. This reduces eye stress and relaxes the mind and body, thereby improving vision.

Treat Sinus Problems for Dry or Watery Eyes

The sinuses must be cleared for proper circulation to the eyes. Both dry and watery eyes are signs of imbalance in the organs. The liver, colon, or kidneys may not be functioning properly, which may cause dry or watery eyes. The eyes are not the cause of eye defects. The eyes only show the effects of what is going on in the internal organs. Pay close attention to your diet. Are you eating too much meat, sugar, fats, and oils or dry baked foods; or too much water, soda, juice, and raw food? Get rid of the cause and the problem will vanish!

Important Eye Health Note: Symptoms of disease, illness, or eye defects are only the effects of deeper causes. Find out what is causing these symptomatic effects. Get rid of the causes, and the effects will cease. The Holy Book says: "The curse causeless, shall not come." Follow the instructions in the diet section and throughout the book to improve your health, and that will in turn improve your vision and mental clarity—healthy body, healthy eyes; unhealthy body, unhealthy eyes.

THINK ON THE THINGS YOU WANT

Dr. Frederick Tilney, who inspired millions of people in the early and mid-1900s, constantly emphasized that "action always follows the thoughts you think—so think on the things you want."

Too many people think that they are worthless, they will never amount to anything in life, they can never be happy, and they feel no one loves them. Is that you talking? It is much better to think that you will be successful and healthy, that you will reach inner peace and happiness, plus achieve the love you want in a harmonious relationship or marriage, and attain perfect eyesight.

To achieve all these things, we are taught by Dr. Tilney to "burn these positive ideas into your mind." See the beautiful and good in people and life. If you look for goodness, you'll find it. Conversely, if you look for bad only, you'll find that too! Be thankful for your life, your health, your possessions, your family and friends. Take nothing for granted. Be grateful for what you have, and you will get more with less struggle and strain.

We have to kill the monster in the ego that wants to be admired—wants everything to go its way at all costs. Get into the habit of forgiving others. Give out words of encouragement and inspiration to yourself and others. We all feel uplifted by an occasional inspirational boost of confidence from a friend, coworker, or family member at the right time.

Depression, moodiness, and melancholy are epidemic in the world today. In Chinese medicine, the liver and gallbladder are seen as the rulers of our moods and vision. A congested, toxic liver can cause anger, frustration, depression, and suicidal tendencies. Anger is stored in the gallbladder. A healthy liver instills kindness, calmness, and perfect eyesight. If anger is present, kindness disappears. Kindness dispels anger. A clean liver gives us clear discernment, good health, and spiritual inspiration. So, start on your liver cleansing program today! Keep the fats, oils, and concentrated sugars down in your diet. Eat plenty of green vegetables, root vegetables, seeds, lean protein or vegetarian protein from hemp, peas, and whole grains. You liver will thank you for it.

HOW TO OVERCOME DISCOURAGEMENT

There is much confusion and negativity in the world today. Via the radio, television, movies, and newspapers, we hear and see nothing but the evils of the world. Rarely do we ever hear truthful answers about solving these problems. And when a good answer is given, it is knocked down by the so-called experts.

If the media doesn't discourage us, our relatives and friends tell us we will not amount to anything. "It's no use trying to improve your eyesight. It can't be done." "Just wear glasses like everyone else." "It takes too much work to improve vision." And on and on. Even our own thoughts tell us "it's impossible, perfect eyesight cannot be achieved." Nothing can ever be accomplished with this negative attitude. The ancient sages teach us not to dwell on the negative side of life. Be positive in whatever you do. Stop listening to those who discourage you from performing your eye exercises. They will say, "you cannot attain perfect eyesight." Instead, in a calm, positive manner, set out to practice the eye and health teachings in this book.

Each day discover new ways to improve your eyesight. Use your intuition or inner vision to give you answers for improved health and clear eyesight. Superior health and clear vision will in turn enhance your insight and intuition about your life, career, and future goals. Lighten up your life, and your life will be full of light. Read spiritual, health, and positive psychology books to help you understand meditation, energy, and your mind, body, and spirit. Follow the example of those who have accomplished great spiritual deeds to help the world understand the nature of existence.

MAGIC FORMULA FOR SUCCESS

If there is a "magic formula" for success and happiness, it is a thankful attitude of mind. An attitude of self-pity and depression is a curse; it paralyzes your thoughts and actions. It stops you from attaining perfect eyesight and inner happiness. Being thankful can lift you out of depression. Success in any endeavor is much easier with a thankful attitude. In fact, thankfulness is considered prayer in the truest sense of the word. If we are thankful all day long, we are in touch with divine order—we are aware, mindful, and respectful of others, nature, and God. We are thankful for our life—our very existence.

Everyone loves to associate with people who are bright, positive, appreciative, and thankful. Begin today to be a positive person. Look for the truth. Be thankful for all the wonderful people and possessions in your life. See the beautiful in everyone and everything. Give yourself words of encouragement. Feel strength, courage, and confidence flowing in your life. This is the real "magic formula for success."

Real success is not about money or material possessions or power over others. Real success and fulfillment in life comes from getting in harmony with the forces of nature and God or Tao. It is being grounded, centered, and balanced. It is deep inner contentment and happiness for just being in the moment during your daily work and activities. Every moment is a celebration of your eternal existence. Make your life constructive and creative. Your divine purpose will then be achieved.

The Empty Mind Technique

Zen and Taoist masters speak about the "empty mind." This is a quiet mind—a rested mind, free from anxiety. We continually pressure and push ourselves to figure out life and its problems. We eventually exhaust our energy and we end up in suffering, frustration, and misery. When we learn to let go of the stress in our mind, body, and emotions, and become internally quiet and peaceful, that's when the answers to the riddle of life come to us. It is this rested state—an awareness of the "Now" or present moment—that gives true inner peace and happiness. Being anxious about the past or future pushes us further away from doing the things we need to do right now.

Let go and just watch. Observe and give attention to what is right in front of you. You will be focused, balanced, centered, and grounded between Heaven and Earth. Then your life will unfold in a harmonious manner. The ancients called this true meditation. We can call this eternal meditation or "Be Here Now" meditation. This is also the secret formula to a calm mind and clear, sharp vision, which is a brain-mind (psycho-spiritual) phenomena.

Persian Sufi Mind-Eye Breathing Technique

This Sufi Breathing technique is known in the Middle East to prevent hair loss, improve vision, and overcome wrinkles. It also helps to stimulate and maintain the thyroid and pituitary glands in perfect working order.

1. In a standing position, place your feet about shoulder width apart.
2. Close the right nostril with your right thumb and inhale deeply through the left nostril until your chest expands fully.
3. Next, close both nostrils with thumb and forefinger, while bending over from the waist, head lowered, knees slightly bent. Hold your breath in this position for 20 to 40 seconds, or as long as comfortable. While in this lowered position, a strong pulsation of blood will be felt in the head, eyes, mouth, tongue, and brain. It will give you a flushed feeling from the chest to the top of the head.
4. Next, slowly straighten up, and let your breath flow out from your right nostril.

If you are ill or have high blood pressure, perform this exercise sitting straight up without bending over. If you are in good health, and you feel a little dizziness or lightheadedness during or after this movement, cut back to only 5 to 10 seconds of holding your breath with your head lowered. Build up to 40 seconds over several weeks. Be persistent, and after a few sessions the dizziness will disappear, and you'll begin to feel elated and energized.

This breathing exercise is designed to burn up toxins and poisons in the body and purify the blood stream, thus imparting a glowing complexion and clear, sharp vision. Always remember to inhale through the left nostril and exhale through the right. To benefit from its full value, perform this exercise no more than 3 times per session, and 3 to 4 times per week, or once every day if you want.

Tranquil Breathing Meditation Technique

When the mind is tranquil, mental clarity and vision automatically improve.

1. Sit straight in a chair. Relax body and mind totally. Just let go. Close your eyes.
2. Next, simply inhale slowly and calmly in and out through the nose—extend the breath for as long as you can on the inhale, and exhale.
3. Visualize tranquillity; go beyond your body sensations, and into serene tranquillity. Perform this Tranquil Breathing meditation technique for 3 to 5 minutes or up to 10 minutes.

If your mind starts drifting and thinking about things, simply place your attention and intention on your breath coming in and out of your nose, until tranquillity is attained. It helps to gaze at the tip of your nose while breathing in and out. The mind will focus more easily at a single point of attention on the breath coming in and out of the nose. Eventually, your breath will become almost automatic.

Once the breathing technique is initiated and tranquillity is reached, the breath or spiritual essence that sustains the physical body will take over. In this state of tranquillity, physical and spiritual healings can take place. You will be in touch with the creative force of the universe. Miracles often happen in this tranquil state, including eyesight improvement and disappearance of disease.

We hope you have enjoyed reading *The Art of Cosmic Vision* as much as we enjoyed writing it for you. We challenge you now to take the next step in your quest for improved vision. That next step is practical application. Any achievement in life requires practice, persistence, and consistency. Natural eyesight training requires the same dedication and discipline as any other goal in life. Dr. Bates said, "Eyesight is your most precious possession." You cannot afford to lose it. Others have perfected their vision, and so can you. Start on your vision-training program today, and enjoy the blessings of perfect eyesight for the rest of your long healthy life!

Write, email, or call us if you have any questions, or tell us of your progress in improving your vision. We would like to hear testimonials from people around the world who have benefited from the teachings presented in *The Art of Cosmic Vision*. Best wishes and blessings in your quest for perfect eyesight and super health.

Appendix

Vision Wisdom from Holistic Health and Natural Eye Specialists

This appendix offers you some pretty amazing secret techniques to improve your vision and to enhance your health and well-being. These "vision secrets" come to us from eye doctors and health specialists from around the world, drawing on traditions dating from early America, as well as the knowledge of ancient cultures of both the West and the East.

EYES REFLECT THE HEALTH OF THE BODY

From Professor Chee Soo

The whites of the eyes reflect the condition of internal health. If there is yellow in the whites of the eyes, liver jaundice is indicated. Constant red eyes reflect a bad liver. A toxic, inflamed liver, according to traditional Chinese medicine, causes one to easily become angry, upset, depressed, and impatient, with reddish eyes.

Professor Chee Soo, a Taoist teacher and writer, says: "A gray or blue 'eye-white' color means that the person is losing their eyesight and may, if these symptoms are ignored, eventually go blind."

Purplish red eyes or eye-whites could be a sign of color blindness. Black indicates kidney problems, green indicates cancer, and brown denotes the presence of stones or cysts. Healthy eyes are clear, steady, and sparkling, without redness, whether the irises are brown, blue, green, or gray. Very little eye-white should be visible. A healthy, vibrant person has more iris than eye-white showing.

CLEAN OUT YOUR BLOODSTREAM AND IMPROVE YOUR VISION
From Benedict Lust, M.D., N.D., D.C., D.O.

Dr. Benedict Lust, an early twentieth-century naturopathic and medical doctor, states: "If your eyesight was nearly normal in your youth, there is no sensible reason why it should not continue in that condition all through your life. Bad eyesight comes from abuse of the eyes through neglect, strain, or the eating of improper foods. All of these causes can be corrected at any time through the utilization of common-sense health methods. The first step is to clean out your bloodstream."

GET FITTED FOR WEAKER LENSES
From optometrists Lowell Rehner and John Ross

Dr. Lowell Rehner and Dr. John Ross are natural eye specialists and graduates from the Northern Illinois College of Optometry. Dr. Ross later taught practical optometry. They both taught natural eyesight training methods to Army and Navy recruits with great success.

They recommended: "Never wear glasses while doing the eye training exercises. If your eyes show but a small amount of error, leave glasses off entirely once you start this treatment. If you must wear glasses in order to pursue your everyday life put them on again after each session of exercising, but, in a week or two, when your sight has markedly improved, visit your eye doctor and get fitted with weaker lenses.

"It may be necessary, in extremely bad cases, to do this several times, over an extended period of time, before your eyes reach their highest point of recovery or until you can dispense with glasses entirely. This, however, is infinitely better than changing to stronger and stronger lenses every few years as would otherwise be the case."

STOP DAYDREAMING!

From Robert Zuraw

"Daydreamers have the pernicious habit of staring out into empty space, blocking out all vision. They usually hold their breath. They prefer not to see reality; fixing their gaze upon an immovable object, which in turn fixes the eye muscles and weakens the sight and eye accommodation. This is a bad habit of nearsighted people. Cut out daydreaming! If you must daydream, then close your eyes."

VISION IS YOUR MOST PRECIOUS POSSESSION

From William H. Bates, M.D.

Dr. William H. Bates, a great pioneer in natural eye training, says this about perfecting vision: "Vision is the most vital of the five senses. The fullest enjoyment of life comes through the eyes—the color of a flower, the form of beauty, the smile of a friend. At work, at home, and at play—most of the things we do lose much of their pleasure without normal vision. You can learn to have good vision throughout life when you learn to use your eyes properly under the conditions modern life imposes upon them."

COMB YOUR HAIR AND IMPROVE YOUR EYESIGHT!

From Yan Shou Shu

Yan Shou Shu, a Chinese health specialist, says: "Frequent combing or brushing the hair can improve vision and dispel bad internal wind or gas. Brushing hair while bent over is helpful for deafness and blurred vision." Try it and see what happens. You might even grow thicker, longer hair.

 ## Distance Vision Exercise: See Like a Telescope with Your Naked Eye

From Edmund Shaftsbury

Edmund Shaftsbury, an early 1900s writer on health and human magnetism, shared the following suggestion derived from the practices of early American Indians.

"The American Indians are known to have the strongest eyes in the world. They have the closest thing to 'telescopic vision.' They can see objects in the far distance that the average person would need a telescope to see.

"Here is an exercise that is similar to the ones the Indians practiced for clear, sharp telescopic vision.

1. Focus your eyes on the tip of your nose for 6 seconds.
2. Next, look at a nearby object, then glance 20 feet further, then 50 feet, 100 feet, 1000 feet, and finish by looking into the horizon. Gently try to see the objects as clearly as possible.

"Repeat this exercise several times for 3–5 minutes, 3 or 4 times a week. Eventually, your vision will become perfectly clear."

STRENGTHEN YOUR STOMACH AND IMPROVE YOUR VISION

From Jethro Kloss

Jethro Kloss, a famous herbalist and author of the classic book *Back to Eden*, states: "Eye troubles are caused mainly from a deranged stomach, for the eyes receive their nourishment from the food taken into the stomach, and naturally the eating of unhealthful foods and drinks such as tea, coffee, salt, alcoholic drinks, tobacco, etc., weakens the nerves and hinders the free circulation to the eyes. Unhealthful foods and drinks cause impure blood and when the circulation carries impure blood to the eyes, it weakens them. The all-important thing is to eat food that will give you a pure blood stream."

HOW TO PREVENT EYESTRAIN AND DEFECTIVE EYES WITH THE ALTERNATE GAZE TECHNIQUE

From W. L. Woodruff

W. L. Woodruff was a writer, lecturer, and physical culturist in the 1930s–'40s. Mr. Woodruff, who had a full head of hair and sharp eyesight into his 80s, says: "Of course there are several reasons for defective eyes, but the chief cause is strain of the fine little muscles, which change the focus or size of the pupil (aperture or iris) on the same principle as in a camera. Also, they cause headaches in some cases.

"While doing tedious work, like accounting or reading, the eye aperture is larger than when looking away at a distance in good light, when the aperture changes and becomes smaller.

"Now, if you keep the eyes in one focus too long, strain results. The remedy is 'Alternate your Gaze'! Here is a good habit to follow, when doing tedious close work or reading: Look away into the distance—the farther away the better. Do this every five or ten minutes. Too much tension in any one position can weaken any muscle in the body, especially delicate eye muscles, nerves, and tiny blood vessels.

"Just try standing in one position too long. It is easier to walk around a long time and benefit the muscles and nervous system because you are alternating the position of the muscles involved.

"In reading or other close work for eyes, alternate the focus by looking at something distant every couple of minutes or so. This helps rest the little muscles that regulate the eye aperture."

LOOK UP FROM YOUR CLOSE WORK
From optometrists Lowell Rehner and John Ross

Drs. Ross and Rehner also place great emphasis on the importance of looking up and away from our close work to avoid eyestrain and tension.

"Look up and away from your close work at frequent intervals. No matter how fascinating or important your reading, drawing, or sewing may be, glance away from it for a second or two every few minutes. This is just as important as it is simple to do.

"If these muscles are kept in a state of contraction for long periods of time without relaxation, they tend to remain cramped when we do finally order them to relax by looking up and away. This is especially true of the muscles of accommodation.

"If you have ever carried a heavy suitcase quite a distance before setting it down, you have noticed how long it takes for your fingers to uncurl. This is because the flexor muscles tend to remain in a state of contraction. The same thing can happen to the accommodative eye muscles when they remain contracted for long periods of time.

"By looking up and away from our close work at frequent intervals we can minimize this muscle cramping which causes the eyes to remain focused for near objects when we wish to see farther away."

DISCOVER DR. PEPPARD'S SECRET TO PREVENT NEARSIGHTEDNESS

From Dr. Harold M. Peppard

Dr. Harold M. Peppard wrote *Sight Without Glasses* in 1940. After giving the warning that "when the print is held too close, myopia (nearsightedness) will be the result," he gives us instructions on how to read properly without straining and weakening our eyes.

- Sit properly. Spine straight. Hold the head balanced over the body—not bending forward.
- Hold the book up toward the eyes, not lazily place it in the lap. Fourteen to sixteen inches is the proper distance for reading.
- Arrange the light. Have plenty of light without glare.
- Read easily and deliberately, word by word. Do not scan and skim. In this fashion, you train your eyes to act normally when they read, and so avoid acquiring abnormal activities.
- Read only when you feel able. When you are sick or tired the eyes, too, are sick and weary, and need your consideration.
- Do not read while eating or after eating for at least one hour.

STRENGTHEN YOUR EYE MUSCLES FOR PERFECT EYESIGHT

From optometrists Lowell Rehner and John Ross

Again, Drs. Ross and Rehner advocate eye muscle exercises to improve eye-focusing power.

"The eye muscles, which have so much to do with the focusing power of the eyes, are the same as other muscles of the body. Disuse weakens them—allows the sight to become stale—proper use strengthens them. Eye muscles need the variety of 'pulls' of diversified focusing intensities. A constant sameness of use is deadening to eye muscles.

"It is only when they are all used properly and enough that they each exert the amount of pull or pressure on the eyeball required to keep it functioning correctly so that the light rays come to an exact focus on the retina. . . . Also, massage the eyelids, which stimulates fresh blood to and around the eyeballs."

Practice the exercises in this book for focusing power.

Exhaling Bull Technique for Eye Power and Rejuvenation

*From Professor Godfrey Rodrigues and
Dr. George Clements*

All animals know instinctively the value of exhalation. You have often heard the horse blowing through its nostrils or a dog panting or sneezing with vigor. Professor Godfrey Rodrigues says in his book *Key to Life:* "What animal has more strength for its size than a bull? When he blows his nostrils, it reacts like a fountain of force.

"The bull knows that the more he exhales, the stronger and stronger he becomes. Continually blowing or exhaling, the larger his chest grows, the smaller his waist becomes, and the more poisonous waste is eliminated from his lungs.

"The Exhaling Bull technique is an excellent exercise given by Dr. George Clements, a natural health doctor and author of many health books.

1. Exhale to the limit, blowing your breath out as long as possible.
2. Increase the exhalation by hard coughing; then hold your breath for a few seconds. This creates a suction in the lungs that draws more poison from the body.
3. Finally blow out the last bit of air. In removing the stale air, we make more room for fresh air. After exhaling, the air comes in effortlessly.

"Foul air lowers our vitality, while fresh air gives us more vim and vigor. You will notice that after a session of 'exhaling,' your eyesight will be clearer and sharper. This encourages you to perform it every day. You finally get the idea of how important this exhaling technique is for relaxing and rejuvenating your eyes, lungs, and health."

 ## Using the Eye-Xerciser
From Gaylord Hauser

The regular use of the Eye-Xerciser will aid in strengthening all of the eye muscles. Hold Eye-Xerciser 5 inches away from your nose (or copy this page and tape it on a wall), with your nose in a direct line with the center spot.

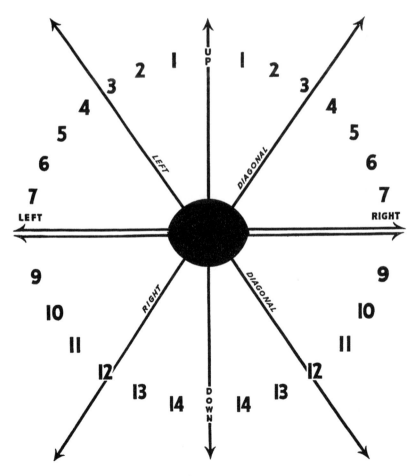

Fig. Appendix 1. Eye-Xerciser

1. Hold your head still and move your eyes on the "up" and "down" arrow 14 times.
2. Let eyes follow the "left" and "right" arrow 14 times.
3. Repeat this process with the "right diagonal" and "left diagonal" arrows 14 times in each direction.
4. Next, make a complete circle to the right, and blink at each number.
5. Repeat procedure counterclockwise.

Perform entire eye exercise 2 or 3 times per week.

TO BLINK OR NOT TO BLINK—THAT IS THE QUESTION!

From Michio Kushi

Michio Kushi, the world's leading exponent of macrobiotics, the founder of the East West Foundation and the Kushi Institute, and author of many books on health and diet, has some interesting things to say about eye-blinking and health: "The standard speed of blinking is three times per minute, or once every twenty seconds. The less blinking the better. Blinking is closing the eyes more, which is a sign of excess yin [water in the body].

"A healthy person's eyes can go without blinking for many minutes; a baby hardly blinks at all. A person who blinks less is currently in a more active sharp condition, in both physical and mental character.

"A person who blinks more than three times per minute is in a state of declining health, due to the consumption of excessive liquid, fruit, and sugar.

"If blinking is abnormally frequent, a person is suffering from nervous disorders and is experiencing extreme sensitivity, fear, and irritability. If we blink more and more we finally close our eyes and die."

Eye-Blinking Linked to Inner Health, Energy, and Personal Magnetism

"We have our best health as babies and young children, provided our parent's diet was good before our birth. Babies are relatively clean and contracted internally. Did you ever notice that babies rarely blink their eyes while awake? Babies also do not show much 'whites' around the iris. Why? Because their cells, tissues, nervous system, and brain are not expanded with yin foods: excess water, sugar, fruit, soda, sugars, coffee, alcohol, drugs, and so on.

"I have observed drug addicts and some people on high yin diets (exclusive raw foods: fruit, vegetables, juices, sprouts, etc.), blinking fifteen to twenty times or more per minute. They are high strung, nervous, oversensitive, super-critical, negative, paranoid, and fearful. One can sense an uneasy tension surrounding them. They show a lot of eye-whites, which indicates an expanded nervous system and excess water retention.

"Healthy magnetic men and women are calm and peaceful. They hardly blink at all. Their faces glow and they have magnetic eyes, with very little eye-whites showing. You don't feel nervous or tense around them. They are positive, creative, and courageous, without paranoia or fear. They see reality, people, and the world with clear insight.

"Excess water or other liquid intake expands the kidneys and bladder, which can lead to water on the brain. The brain, like a camera, records pictures taken in through the eyes. Our eyes are like the aperture of a camera.

"Excess water in the body cells and brain causes one to blink involuntarily in an effort to rid the body of excess water (yin). Blinking more does not lubricate the eyes, the eye muscles, eye nerves, or tear duct glands. Excess blinking is the result of excess mucus and watery lubrication in the eyes and body tissues.

"When you are healthy, fit, rested, calm, and peaceful, you need not worry about blinking—your body will take care of that task for you. A healthy person blinks two or three times a minute. More blinking only shows internal imbalance and poor health. Chinese Natural Medicine teaches us that excess blinking also indicates a weak expanded (yin) liver, a major cause of nearsightedness (myopia).

"Observe people in your surroundings. Put this knowledge to the acid test. Watch for signs, symptoms, and characteristics in yourself and others. Knowledge without practical experience is useless. Above all, observe yourself. Are you blinking excessively? Are you myopic or farsighted? Is your health below par? Energy low? Fatigue high? Why? Keep digging and answers will be given to you. Knock and the door shall be opened. Ask and you shall receive. After all, it is your own health and vision! Why not do something to improve your health and vision today?"

DIET AND DO-IN HEALTH DIAGNOSIS THROUGH THE EYES

From Jean Rofidal

Jean Rofidal, writing in *DO-IN: Eastern Massage and Yoga Techniques*, draws a close link between the health of the body organs and eye health:

"The eyes have a close connection with the liver and when the liver is functioning badly the eyes ache. When a person has eaten too much or had a meal that is yin (sweets, alcohol) the eyes are tired and have circles around them and do not bear the light very well.

"Our eyes betray our thoughts, good or bad, and our kindness or unkindness.

"In women the eyes are linked with the ovaries and in men with the testicles. Sexual excess is revealed by black circles around the eyes. In men, the eyes should be small and almond-shaped. In women, they should be bigger and rounder (yin).

"If the kidneys are overworked by too much drink, especially alcohol, the eyes become tired and sensitive and the puffy lower eyelids form 'bags' under the eyes. A further pouch can form under the first; it indicates a degeneration of the intestines. It is often seen in the elderly."

HEED THE WARNING

Soybeans, Soy Oil, Tofu Linked to Thyroid Problems, Protruding Eyes, Liver Disease, and Weak Immunity

From Naboru Muramoto

Naboru Muramoto, a leading macrobiotic teacher and author of *Healing Ourselves*, states: "Soybeans are not recommended as a bean dish, despite their protein content. [Soybeans are not a building protein—at best they are a low-maintenance protein and very difficult to digest.]

"The soy protein contains a certain harmful acid, which can be eliminated only by elaborate [and long] cooking methods. This is why Orientals usually eat soybeans in the form of tofu, a sort of 'soybean cheese.' But, to make it less harmful and digestible, tofu must be baked or sautéed until it is hard. This takes out the sticky substance in the fat. Soy products make the blood sticky and weaken liver function, which lowers red blood cell count and depresses the immune system."

However, tofu is not desirable either. Protruding eyes [thyroid malfunction] are often a sign of a large consumption of soybeans. This also goes for tempeh, soy dogs, soy oil, soy burgers, and soy margarine. Obtain your protein from a variety of other beans and legumes. They are easier and quicker to prepare and taste better too, without all the health-damaging side effects.

GOOD EYE NUTRITION

From Chris D. Meletis and Wayne Centrone

In their article, "Retinopathy and Macular Degeneration," *Alternative and Complementary Therapies* 8, no. 2 (2004), the authors recommend: organic foods, super-food supplements, spirulina, alfalfa, chlorella, blue-green algae, nutritional yeast, acidophilus, ginkgo 160 mg, coQ10 (50–150 mg divided doses), vitamin E 400–800 IU, vitamin A (fish oil) 10,000 IU, black currant seed oil for omega-3 essential fatty acids, lutein 10–20 mg, quercetin (400 mg, 4 x day), selenium 200 mcg, rutin 1,000 mg, alpha lipoic acid 500–900 mg, magnesium 350 mg, bioflavonoids 1,000 mg, bilberry 200–480 mg, melatonin 200 mcg 2–3 hours before bed; milk thistle, 2–4 capsules daily.

ANCIENT ZEN-TAOIST TECHNIQUE TO REDUCE SWOLLEN EYES
From Master Da Liu

Taoist Master Da Liu wrote in his *Taoist Health Exercise Book:* "If blood circulation is poor, your feet will be cold, since this area is farthest away from the center of the body. A great Confucian scholar believed strongly in rubbing the feet (bottom and top of feet). He proved that swelling of the eyelids could be completely relieved by rubbing the feet every day two hundred times. If you do this exercise every day, it can prevent fever of the inner organs."

 ## Eye Power-Gaze Technique
From O. Everett Hughes, N.D.

Here is a simple but powerful eye technique that can be performed quickly and easily at any time. O. Everett Hughes, N.D., writing in *Natural Health Guardian* (February 1958) said: "I wore glasses for years, but after taking these exercises for a year, optometrists told me I did not need glasses."

1. Close one eye tight. Put more power to it, trying to shut it tighter. Squeeze the eye hard, while shut. Go easy the first few times.
2. Now change to the other eye and do the same with it.
3. Then, with both eyes, look hard at some object straight ahead. Look at the object very hard. Put power behind the look.

4. Then look hard to one corner, but keep facing ahead. Just turn the eyes. Put pressure behind that look.

5. Now change and look to the other corner. Remember, don't turn your head.

Do this "hard look" exercise to all corners of the eye. If you notice any soreness, you can put a little more pressure in that direction.

 ## Secret of the Steady Eye Technique
From Professor Robert B. Hagmann

Professor Robert B. Hagmann, a well-known natural eye specialist in the early 1950s, gives us his secret to perfect eyesight in the Steady Eye technique:

"Understand, our eyes work exactly like a camera; move or jerk the camera and the picture becomes distorted. A moving eye also distorts the vision. We must learn to hold our eyes with steadiness.

"During the odd moments of the day, practice keeping your eyes still, striving not to move them in the least; relax and breathe naturally. Do not hold your breath. Do not frown or make faces; keep the face relaxed; while keeping the eyes as still as possible.

"Your eyes may 'tear' during this practice; don't be alarmed, just let the tears flow down the cheeks. It's only the eyes shifting back to their normal position. While maintaining the steady gaze, also pay attention to the side areas [peripheral vision]."

NATUROPATHIC CURE FOR WEAK EYESIGHT
From Benedict Lust, M.D., N.D., D.C., D.O.

In the early 1900s Dr. Benedict Lust, the well-known holistic doctor, wrote many books and articles on health, diet, eyes, and natural healing. The following is from his informative articles on improving weak eyesight:

"To cure poor eyesight means to restore it so that objects are focused right, so that the eyesight is 100% again. In many cases, glasses can be dispensed with and eyes made to see again by correcting the shape of the eyeball. This is accomplished in the following way.

"The eyeball is the place of attachment of eight muscles, which pull the eye up, down, to the side, and toward the nose. Like all muscles, these may be either strong or weak. If one or another is stronger than the rest, the muscle will pull the eyeball out of shape.

"Thus, a good proportion of poor eyesight is due to weak eye muscles. The cure lies in making the weak muscles strong and firm again. Eye exercises strengthen the eye muscles safely and eye gymnastics are a satisfactory and productive treatment."

Dr. Lust's Eye Gymnastics

Part I

The following are simple and efficient eye gymnastics. Perform each exercise twenty times.

1. Roll the eyes up. Try to look at the top of your head.
2. Roll the eyes down, try to look at your bottom teeth.
3. Look out of the right corner of both eyes. Roll the eyes to the right side.
4. Look out of the left side of the eyes. Roll the eyes to the left.
5. Roll the eyeballs around, in a circle; look up, right side, down, left side. Look at every corner, ceiling, and floor of the room you are sitting in, without moving your head.
6. Look at the tip of your nose; make yourself cross-eyed.

⟳ Part II

Tired eyes, in many cases, become congested with blood, due to strain, too much close work, or weak eye muscles. Eyes can be toned up, blood circulation improved, and blood vessels strengthened by practicing these eye-care techniques regularly.

1. Close the eyelids, press the eyeballs gently into the socket, hold and count 10. Release. Repeat 10 times.
2. Dip a cloth into cold water. Close eyelids and put the cold compress to the eyes. Repeat.
3. Close eyelids. With tips of fingers gently placed against skin over eyes, circle the fingers rapidly, barely touching the eyelids. This is a very relaxing eye-beauty treatment.

Important Eye Training Note: Practice these eye gymnastic exercises no more than twice a week for best results. Close your eyes and Palm 10 minutes after each eye exercise session.

ORIENTAL MEDICINE AND EYE HEALTH
From Beverly Brough

An article by Beverly Brough, "Who Needs Glasses?" in the *East-West Journal,* August 1980, states: "Oriental medicine goes one step further in seeing good vision as part of total health. In the five transformations theory, eyesight falls under the element wood and therefore is connected with the liver, so those foods that affect the liver would also affect vision. Foods that are especially damaging to the liver are chemicals, sugar, alcohol, cold drinks, oily [fatty] food, and general overeating. These foods as well as [too much] fruits and too much liquid cause the eyeball to bulge. When the eyeball is elongated in this manner, nearsightedness results. Farsightedness is caused by a shrinking of the eyeball, due to an excess of meats [and yang spicy foods].

"One treatment for getting rid of excess liquid in the eyes is to put a few drops of light sesame oil in each eye before bed. Heat the oil almost to a boil, then cool to room temperature and strain through cheesecloth before dropping in the eyes. Sesame oil repels the liquid, which is then discharged out of the eye. Splash with warm salt water in the morning. Try this for three nights in a row.

"Another method to free up liquid in the eyes is to grasp first the upper lids between thumb and first finger and vibrate rapidly. Do the same with the lower lids. You will be able to hear the liquid as it is released from around the eye."

MACROBIOTIC LIVER DIAGNOSIS: YOUR EYES MONITOR THE HEALTH OF YOUR LARGEST ORGAN

From Bill Tims

Bill Tims, macrobiotic teacher, wrote an article entitled "The Liver" in *Bodyhealth: A Guide to Keeping Your Body Well,* an *East-West Journal* anthology published in 1985.

"For the purpose of diagnosis, we can divide . . . liver conditions into two main categories: an overly tight and contracted (yang) condition of the liver and an overly swollen (yin) liver condition.

"First let's . . . determine which of these two liver conditions is likely to arise due to constitutional or inherited tendencies. In traditional [Chinese] medicine, the liver has been associated with the eyes due to their simultaneous embryological development as well as to their connection via the energy meridians of acupuncture. If the eyes are small or tend to cross, if they are close-set, or if the eyebrows grow closely together or slant upward, there is a constitutional tendency for the liver to develop problems from becoming overly contracted. If the eyes are large or tend to move outward or if the eyes are set far apart, there will be more of a tendency for the liver to become swollen. In addition, any inherited or congenital eye defects will usually indicate some related weakness in the liver.

". . . most important in determining the present liver condition, is a thorough assessment of the eyes. If yellow, fatty excess accumulates in the whites of the eyes, this shows a similar fat accumulation in the liver. (This often will ooze or crust [kapha (water) body type], in the corners of the eyes, particularly during sleep when the liver does most of its cleansing of fats from the blood.) If the eyes are red or bloodshot [pitta (fire) body type] or if a rash or inflammation arises between the eyes, this suggests a swollen and inflamed liver condition. The eyes or eyelids or the area between the eyes also . . . develop red spots or stys, a sign of excessive storage of animal protein in the liver.

"If the eyes become watery or swollen or begin to burn or itch, this indicates an overly swollen liver . . . dryness [vata (air) body type] indicates an overly contracted condition. If there appears a single, deep vertical line between the eyes, the liver is overly contracted [yang]; and if there are several shallow vertical lines, the liver is overly expanded [yin]. Crossed eyes, downturned eyes, and farsightedness all indicate a contracted liver condition; eyes drifting outward and upward, as well as nearsightedness, all indicate an expanded liver condition.

"A contracted liver condition is caused by an excessive consumption of meat, eggs, cheese, and baked goods, while an expanded liver condition is caused more by an excessive consumption of drugs, stimulants, alcohol . . . citrus fruits, refined sugar, vinegar, fats, dairy, and oil.

". . . most people have serious health problems resulting from some combination of these foods. In order to restore balance and revive the liver . . . increase your consumption of whole cereal grains and beans, and . . . eat fresh and lightly cooked green leafy vegetables."

CATARACT STUDIES INDICATING SUPPLEMENTS THAT MAY IMPROVE YOUR VISION

From website: i-care.net/eyeresearch.html#cataract

For cataracts, we suggest that you refer to the nutritional recommendations given on the website, *Preventing Blindness through Nutritional*

Intervention, which provides a summary of nutritional eye research. In general, for the prevention of cataract, they support the avoidance of smoking and the use of vitamins A, C, and E, as well as carotene, niacin, riboflavin, and thiamine, procyanidins, alpha lipoic acid, taurine, lutein, cryptoxanthin, and selenium.

IMPROVE YOUR VISION BY BAREFOOT WALKING IN THE WATER, ON THE BEACH, OR ON THE GRASS
From Bernard Jensen, D.C.

World health educator Dr. Bernard Jensen, author of many books on colon therapy, iridology, and health rejuvenation, recommends walking in a bed of sand, with cold water up to your ankles. Walking barefoot in the grass is also very effective.

Dr. Jensen says: "Persons with poor circulation in the lower extremities put an extra burden upon the heart. When there is but slight muscular contraction in the lower extremities, blood is not properly returned to the heart, and leg disorders may develop. To remedy this condition, we devised at the sanitarium . . . the sand walk.

"Every morning we wet down a bed of sand with cold water and patients walked in this cold sand. This massaged the bottoms of their feet and developed the small muscles in their feet and legs. One of the first comments usually made by these patients was that as a result of these sand walks they had warm feet when going to bed at night, whereas never before had they gone to bed with warm feet. The Kneipp grass walk, as used in sanitariums in Germany, is another excellent means of increasing circulation in the lower extremities.

"I have noticed changes in patients using the sand walk or the grass walk that are hard to believe. In most cases the whole body responds when we build strong healthy feet; organs are reflex[ive]ly released.

Eye conditions improve almost immediately. In fact, I have seen eyes improve to such an extent that glasses were no longer needed."

How to Improve Distant Vision Using "Positive Lens" Glasses

From Donald S. Rehm

In the early 1900s a few eye doctors gave their clients "positive lens" glasses to help overcome nearsightedness (myopia). The nearsighted clients who had 20–100 vision or less obtained excellent results with the use of positive lens eyeglasses. Although positive lens glasses are usually given to those who have weak close vision, in this case, they are used to help nearsighted people see better in the distance. Here's a short explanation of how to use the positive lens glasses, from *The Myopia Myth* by Donald S. Rehm (published by the International Myopia Prevention Association, R.D. 5, Box 171, Ligonier, PA 15658).

"Go to a discount store and purchase three pairs of positive lens glasses of three different strengths: +1.00, +2.00, and +3.00. Look on the eyeglass lens for the number, which indicates its strength. These glasses typically sell for only a few dollars.

1. Begin by using the +1.00 lens glasses. Sit in outdoor or bright indoor lighting. Hold a printed page in front of your eyes, and move it to a distance where you can see it clearly.
2. Trace a letter on the page with your eyes; next, close eyes for 10 seconds and relax.
3. Open your eyes while inhaling a gentle breath and gaze at the same letter.
4. Move print 1 inch further away from your eyes and repeat the above steps.
5. Continue to move the print further away in 1-inch increments, as long as you are able to still read the letter. If the print becomes too blurry, move printed page back to where you can read it without strain.

"Do not be in a hurry to improve your vision with this exercise. Make sure you can see the letter clearly before moving the print another inch away from your eyes. For example, if you can only see clearly with your eyes 11 inches away from the print, stay with this distance until the print becomes clear, then move it to 12 inches.

"The ultimate goal of this exercise (using +1.00 lens glasses) is to be able to read the print clearly at least 20 inches away from your eyes. After you succeed with this lens, change to your +2.00 lens glasses. And finally, when you can see the print 20 inches with the +2.00 lens, change to the +3.00 lens glasses and work your way to the 20-inch mark.

"When you can easily see the printed page at 12 inches away from your eyes while using the +3.00 lens glasses, you will have obtained 20–20 vision. At 20 inches away with the +3.00 lens glasses, you'll be seeing much better than 20–20."

Practice this exercise 2 to 3 times per week, for 15 minutes each session. Finish your session by Palming your eyes for 5 minutes. Do not overexercise your eyes. Vision improves faster when eye exercises are performed moderately. When performing this technique with other nearsighted exercises in this book, do not go over 1 hour per eye session total. Use your good judgment on the exercises that best fit your eye condition.

The Art of Reading

From William H. Bates, M.D.

"When reading, you should look at the white spaces between the lines and not directly at the lines themselves. The reason for this is that it is no effort to sweep the eyes over a plain background. Fixing the eyes on individual words and letters involves strain, and strain impairs vision. When a person with normal sight regards the white spaces with a sweeping shift across the page from margin to margin, he can read easily, rapidly, and without fatigue.

"If the same person looks at the letters, the eyes grow tired and the vision becomes poor.

"People who cannot read well at the near point always tend to fix their attention on the print. Consequently their vision becomes worse. Improvement cannot take place until they learn to look at the white spaces between the lines. Reading can be improved by improving the power to remember or imagine whiteness. This improvement can be achieved in the following way.

1. Close your eyes and imagine something even whiter than the page before you, such as: white snow, white starch, white linen.
2. Open your eyes again. If your mental images of whiteness have been clear and intense, you will find that the white spaces between the lines will appear whiter than they really are for a few moments.
3. Repeat this process as a regular drill.

"When your imagination of whiteness has become so good that you can constantly see the spaces between lines as whiter than they really are, the print will seem blacker by contrast and the eye will find itself reading easily and without effort or fatigue. When the imagination of whiteness has reached its maximum intensity, it often happens that one can see a thin white line much better than the rest of the white space. This white line may be compared to a neon light moving swiftly from one margin to the other, immediately under the letters.

"Consciousness of this thin white line is a great help in reading, as it increases the speed both of the eyes and of the mind. Once this illusion of the white line is seen, imagined, or remembered, unlimited reading without fatigue becomes possible."

Ayurvedic Nasal Wash for Clear Vision
From Swami Devi Dayal and the Yoga-Ratnakara

For thousands of years ayurvedic medicine from India has taught the importance of cleansing the nasal passageways to clear the sinus cavities and to attain 20–20 clear vision and beyond! They recommend using a neti pot, a little ceramic pot that holds about 10 to 12 ounces of water. The neti pot has a 3-inch slender nozzle attached to one end to insert into the nose. The neti pot is unsurpassed in cleansing the entire sinus cavity, which helps to clear up sinus congestion, colds, and mucus, which can all create poor vision. Frequent use of the neti pot can help your vision stay clear and sharp.

Swami Devi Dayal of India has this to say about the healing effects of the Nasal Wash: "The Nasal Wash helps to relieve nasal congestion in a few days or weeks. Pyorrhea can be cured in a month or two. Hearing and eyesight are greatly improved in three months. It helps stammering in two months. It strengthens the nerves, clears pimples. Memory is improved. One sleeps deeper and sounder. Snoring is diminished. Migraine headaches are relieved. Mental problems helped. It also helps to prevent and overcome TB, asthma, fevers, and so on.

1. Fill a neti pot (which can be purchased at a health food store) with purified lukewarm water and add about ¼ teaspoon of sea salt.
2. Next, tilt your head down low over a sink to the right (face is pointing toward your left shoulder) and insert the neti pot nozzle into your left nostril. Let the water pour into the left nostril *slowly*. The water will pour out of the right nostril.
3. Repeat the same procedure with the opposite nostril over the sink.
4. Next, tilt your head backward and let the water flow up your right nostril so it runs into your mouth; then spit it out. With your head in this backward position, close the opposite nostril with your finger, so the water will go into the mouth.
5. Repeat with the left nostril.

"For optimum health benefits it is recommended to practice the Neti Pot Nasal Wash daily for a few weeks."

Here is some deep wisdom from the Yoga-Ratnakara, a treatise on ayurvedic medicine: "A person who regularly drinks water through the nose, in the early morning and at night, becomes intelligent, develops eyesight as acute as an eagle, prevents graying hair and wrinkling of skin, and is freed from all diseases."

This is a powerful statement indeed! However, yogis who practice the Nasal Wash technique, along with other physical and spiritual disciplines, are known for their superb health, tranquility, and longevity. It is worth giving it a try for a few weeks, and finding out for yourself whether you can avoid nagging colds, brain fog, and sinus and eye problems.

Chinese Taoist Secret Longevity Eye Exercise

From Master Da Liu

This is a secret eye technique taught by long-lived Taoist masters from the mountains of China. These sages never lose their vision and they are reportedly over one hundred years young and as spry as spring chickens! Master Da Liu, a Tai Chi master from China, lived to 100, and taught these practices to his many students in New York City for 30 years.

1. Sit up with your back straight. Close your eyes. With your first two finger pads, press lightly on the closed eyelids:
2. Inhale gently, hold your breath, and move your eyes 3 times up and down. Exhale. Take a deep breath and relax. Repeat again.
3. Inhale gently. Hold your breath, and move eyes 3 times sideways. Exhale. Take a deep breath and relax. Repeat again.
4. Inhale gently. Hold your breath. Move eyes in a clockwise direction 3 times. Exhale. Take a deep breath and relax. Repeat again.
5. Inhale gently. Hold your breath. Move eyes in a counterclockwise direction 3 times. Exhale. Take a deep breath and relax. Repeat again.

While performing the eye movement, gently press your fingers on your closed eyelids. The value of this special eye exercise lies in combining massage (pressing the closed eyelids with your fingers), deep breathing, and eye exercise movement simultaneously. You can also press your palm on the closed eyelids while performing this technique.

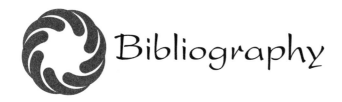# Bibliography

Bates, William H., M.D. *Perfect Sight Without Glasses*. New York: Central Fixation Publishing, 1920.

Chaney, Earlyne. *The Eyes Have It*. York Beach, Maine: Samuel Weiser, 1987.

Chia, Mantak. *Chi Self-Massage: The Taoist Way of Rejuvenation*. Rochester, Vt.: Destiny Books, 2006.

Corbett, Margaret D. *Help Yourself to Better Sight*. New York: Prentice-Hall, 1949.

G.M.Z. Productions. *The Eye Improvement System*. New York: Home Video, 1990.

Gvoquan, Yang. *Three-Bath Qi Gong*. Hong Kong: Hai Feng Publishing, 1989.

Leviton, Richard. *Better Vision in Thirty Days*. Boca Raton, Fla.: Globe Communications, 1994.

Peppard, Harold M. *Sight Without Glasses*. Garden City, N. Y.: Blue Ribbon Books, 1940.

Revien, Leon, O.D., and Mark Gabor. *Sports-Vision*. New York: Workman Publishing, 1981.

Richardson, Dr. R. A. *Strong Healthy Eyes Without Glasses*. Kansas City, Mo.: Eyesight and Health Association Publishers, 1925.

Rofidal, Jean. *DO-IN: Eastern Massage and Yoga Techniques*. Wellingborough, Northamptonshire, England: Thorson Publishers, 1981.

Ross, Dr. John R., and Dr. Lowell Rehner. *The Complete Eye Exercises for the Strengthening and Correction of Defective Eyesight*. Plymouth, Mich.: Hall Publishing, 1943.

Rotte, Joanna, Ph.D., and Koji Yamamoto. *Vision: A Holistic Guide to Healing the Eyesight.* Tokyo: Japan Publications, 1986.

Shaftsbury, Edmund. *Instantaneous Personal Magnetism.* Meriden, Conn.: Ralston University Press, 1926.

Svoboda, Robert E. *Prakruti: Your Ayurvedic Constitution.* Albuquerque, N. Mex.: Geocom, 1988.

Vision WorkOut. *Vision Workout.* Reno, Nev.: Home Video.

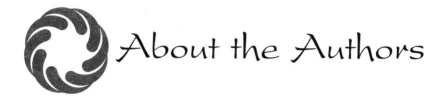 # About the Authors

MASTER MANTAK CHIA

Mantak Chia has been studying the Taoist approach to life since childhood. His mastery of this ancient knowledge, enhanced by his study of other disciplines, has resulted in the development of the Universal Tao System, which is now being taught throughout the world.

Mantak Chia was born in Thailand to Chinese parents in 1944. When he was six years old, he learned from Buddhist monks how to sit and "still the mind." While in grammar school he learned traditional Thai boxing, and soon went on to acquire considerable skill in Aikido, Yoga, and Tai Chi. His studies of the Taoist way of life began in earnest when he was a student in Hong Kong, ultimately leading to his mastery of a wide variety of esoteric disciplines, with the guidance of several masters, including Master I Yun, Master Meugi, Master Cheng Yao Lun, and Master Pan Yu. To better understand the mechanisms behind healing energy, he also studied Western anatomy and medical sciences.

Master Chia has taught his system of healing and energizing practices to tens of thousands of students and trained more than two thousand instructors and practitioners throughout the world. He has established centers for Taoist study and training in many countries around the globe. In June of 1990, he was honored by the International Congress of Chinese Medicine and Qi Gong (Chi Kung), which named him the Qi Gong Master of the Year.

ROBERT LEWANSKI

Robert Lewanski studied the Natural Hygiene System of Health, Diet, and Fasting in 1972, under the direct supervision of Dr. Herbert M. Shelton and Dr. Virginia Vetrano, at Dr. Shelton's Health School in San Antonio, Texas. He was certified in Foot Reflexology by Dr. William Kenner, Dearborn, Michigan, in 1973. From 1975 to 1976, he studied and graduated with high honors from Career Academy, School of Famous TV and Radio Broadcasters, in Washington, D.C. In 1985, he studied Flying Crane Chi Kung Yoga with Dr. Shen Wang and was certified in Chinese Medical Massage by Dr. Wang in 1988.

Lewanski has studied and practiced Du-In self-healing massage, acupressure, Swedish massage, cranial-facial massage, and Shiatsu Oriental massage for twenty years. He has been certified as an Ayurvedic Counselor in Nutrition and Health through the Ayurvedic Institute, Albequerque, New Mexico, by Dr. Vasant Lad, Director, and Dr. Robert Svoboda, Chief Instructor. He has also studied Sun-Do meditation, Chinese Five-Element Nutritional Body Typing, and Taoist Chi Kung Yoga with Master Hyunoong Sunim from Korea.

He is the director of Health Force Center, Royal Oak, Michigan. In addition to being a Chi Kung practitioner and consultant, noted palmist, character reader, and personal fitness trainer, he is also a certified Organic Food Gardener. He served as president of the Detroit chapter of the National Health Federation from 1977 to 1979 and appeared on the J. P. McCarthy Show, WJR, in 1985 and the Dick Purtan Show in 1990.

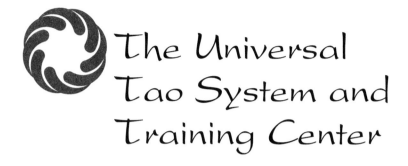

The Universal Tao System and Training Center

THE UNIVERSAL TAO SYSTEM

The ultimate goal of Taoist practice is to transcend physical boundaries through the development of the soul and the spirit within the human. That is also the guiding principle behind the Universal Tao, a practical system of self-development that enables individuals to complete the harmonious evolution of their physical, mental, and spiritual bodies. Through a series of ancient Chinese meditative and internal energy exercises, the practitioner learns to increase physical energy, release tension, improve health, practice self-defense, and gain the ability to heal him- or herself and others. In the process of creating a solid foundation of health and well-being in the physical body, the practitioner also creates the basis for developing his or her spiritual potential by learning to tap into the natural energies of the sun, moon, earth, stars, and other environmental forces.

The Universal Tao practices are derived from ancient techniques rooted in the processes of nature. They have been gathered and integrated into a coherent, accessible system for well-being that works directly with the life force, or chi, that flows through the meridian system of the body.

Master Chia has spent years developing and perfecting techniques for teaching these traditional practices to students around the world

189

through ongoing classes, workshops, private instruction, and healing sessions, as well as books and video and audio products. Further information can be obtained at www.universal-tao.com.

THE UNIVERSAL TAO TRAINING CENTER

The Tao Garden Resort and Training Center in northern Thailand is the home of Master Chia and serves as the worldwide headquarters for Universal Tao activities. This integrated wellness, holistic health, and training center is situated on eighty acres surrounded by the beautiful Himalayan foothills near the historic walled city of Chiang Mai. The serene setting includes flower and herb gardens ideal for meditation, open-air pavilions for practicing Chi Kung, and a health and fitness spa.

The center offers classes year round, as well as summer and winter retreats. It can accommodate two hundred students, and group leasing can be arranged. For information worldwide on courses, books, products, and other resources, see below.

RESOURCES

Universal Healing Tao Center
274 Moo 7, Luang Nua, Doi Saket, Chiang Mai, 50220 Thailand
Tel: (66)(53) 495-596 Fax: (66)(53) 495-852
E-mail: universaltao@universal-tao.com
Web site: www.universal-tao.com

For information on retreats and the health spa, contact:
Tao Garden Health Spa & Resort
E-mail: info@tao-garden.com, taogarden@hotmail.com
Web site: www.tao-garden.com

Good Chi • Good Heart • Good Intention

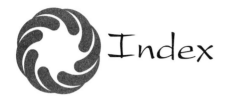

Index

Page numbers in *italics* refer to illustrations.

BOOKS OF RELATED INTEREST

Chi Self-Massage
The Taoist Way of Rejuvenation
by Mantak Chia

Iron Shirt Chi Kung
by Mantak Chia

The Six Healing Sounds
Taoist Techniques for Balancing Chi
by Mantak Chia

Chi Nei Tsang
Chi Massage for the Vital Organs
by Mantak Chia

Cosmic Fusion
The Inner Alchemy of the Eight Forces
by Mantak Chia

Fusion of the Five Elements
Meditations for Transforming Negative Emotions
by Mantak Chia

Fusion of the Eight Psychic Channels
Opening and Sealing the Energy Body
by Mantak Chia

Living in the Tao
The Effortless Path of Self-Discovery
by Mantak Chia and William U. Wei

Inner Traditions • Bear & Company
P.O. Box 388
Rochester, VT 05767
1-800-246-8648
www.InnerTraditions.com

Or contact your local bookseller